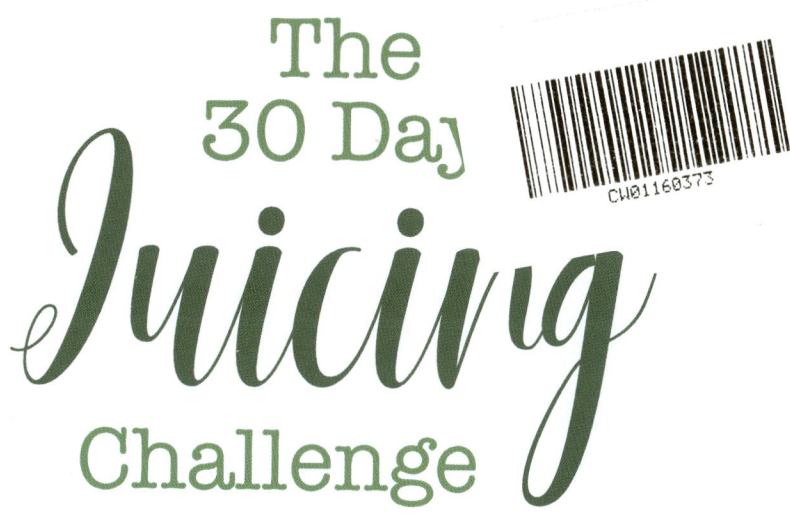

# The 30 Day Juicing Challenge

*One juice a day can change your life!*

*Written and photographed by*

## TRACEE SLOAN

Juicing expert and weight loss coach for juicerecipes.com

Cover photo by Nick Schrader

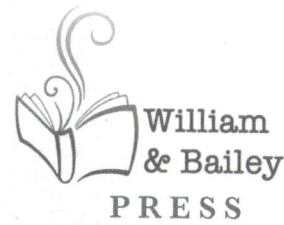

William & Bailey PRESS

First published in 2021 by William & Bailey Press

Copyright © Tracee Sloan

All rights reserved. No part of this publication may be reproduced or distributed in any form or by any means, electronic or mechanical, or stored in a database or retrieval system, without prior written permission from the publisher.

ISBN 978-0-578-98231-1 (Custom Universal)

This book is for entertainment purposes. The publisher and author of this book are not responsible in any manner whatsoever for any adverse effects arising directly or indirectly as a result of the information provided in this book.

Printed in the USA

Front Cover and Page 87-88 Photography: Nick Schrader

Nama J2 Cold Press Juicer Photography: Audrey Ma

Food and Juice Photography: Tracee Sloan

Front and Back Photo Cover Design: Joan Briand and Tracee Sloan

Set Styling: Tracee Sloan

Book Design: Tracee Sloan and Joan Briand

Original Art: Tracee Sloan

## Disclaimer

The opinions expressed in this book are for educational and informational purposes only. They are not intended as a substitute for professional medical advice, diagnosis and treatment. Please consult a physician or other health care professional for your specific health care or medical needs or concerns. The information in this book is not intended to substitute for consultations with your doctor for any health condition.

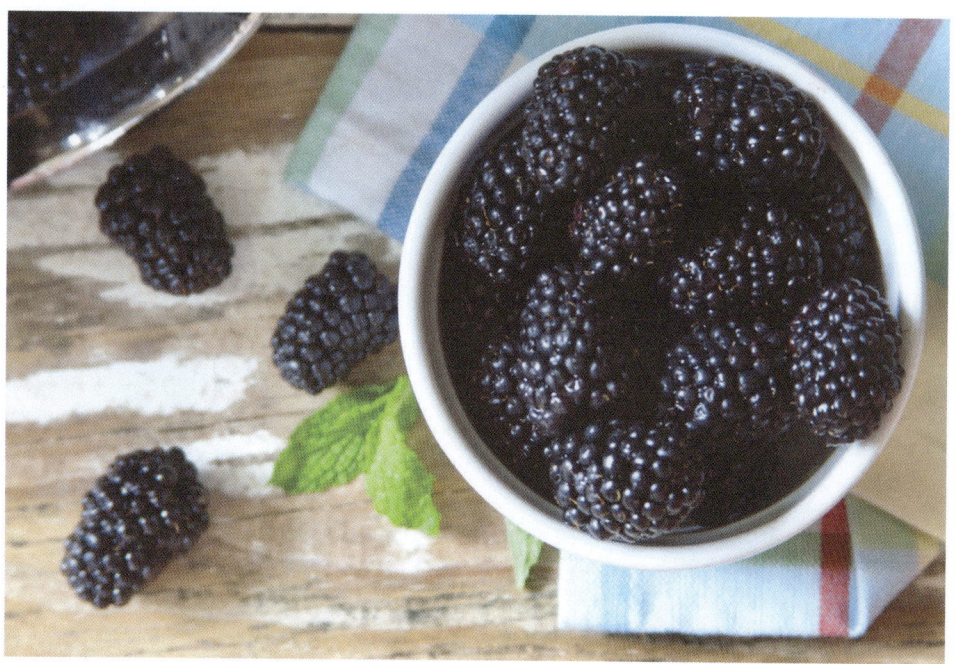

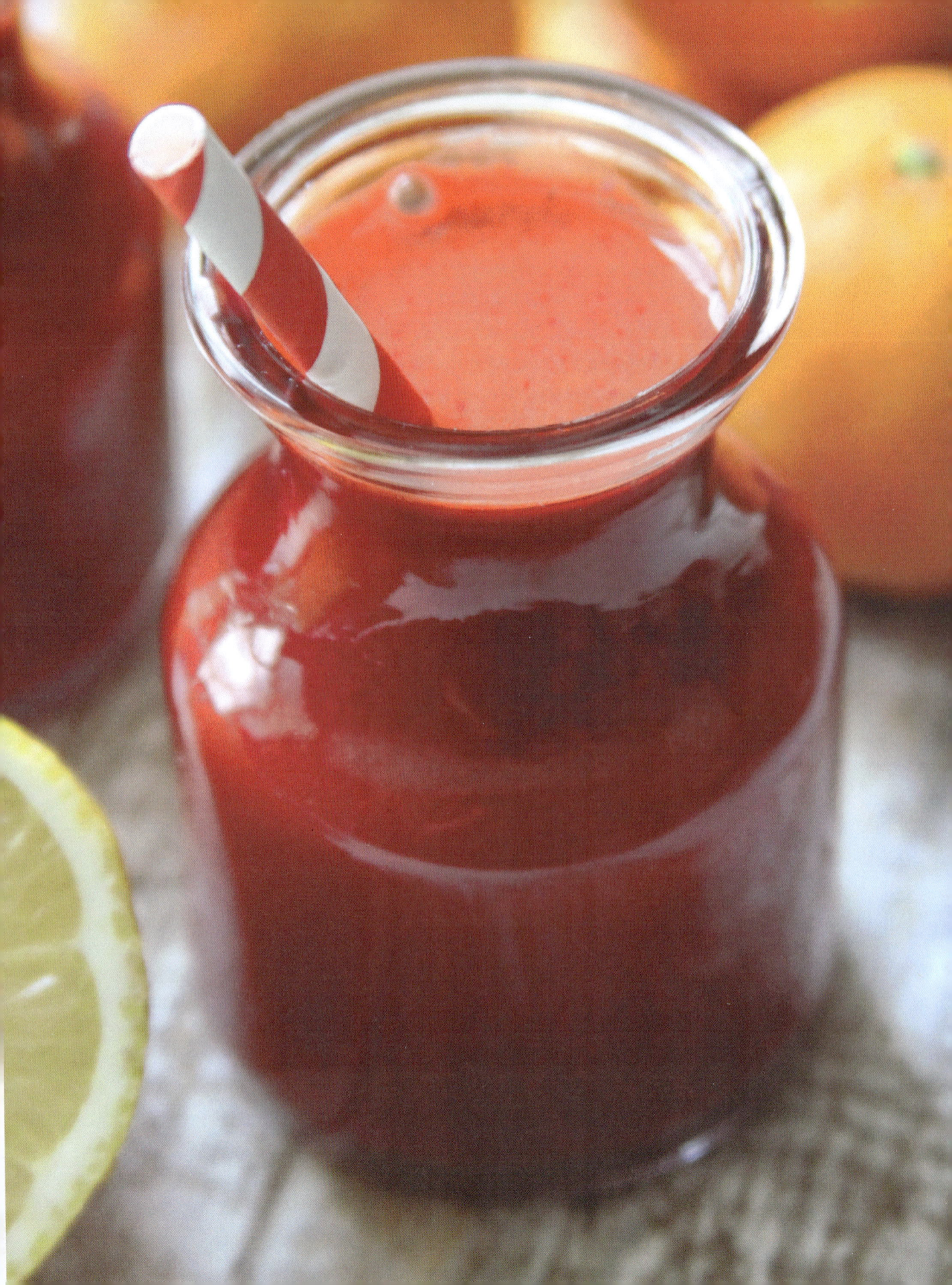

# CONTENTS

| | |
|---|---|
| Succeeding at Your Challenge | 7 |
| *From Visualization to Motivation* | 8 |
| *Why Your Juicer Matters* | 10 |
| *Tips for Cleaning Your Juicer* | 14 |
| *Tips for Storing Your Juice* | 16 |
| *Creating a Juicing Habit* | 18 |
| *The Challenge Tracker* | 20 |
| The 30 Day Challenge | 22 |
| *Days 1-7* | 24 |
| *Days 8-14* | 38 |
| *Days 15-21* | 52 |
| *Days 22-28* | 66 |
| *Days 29-30* | 80 |
| Bonus Recipes | 86 |
| Substitutions for Fruits and Veggies | 94 |
| Resources | 104 |
| About the Author | 105 |

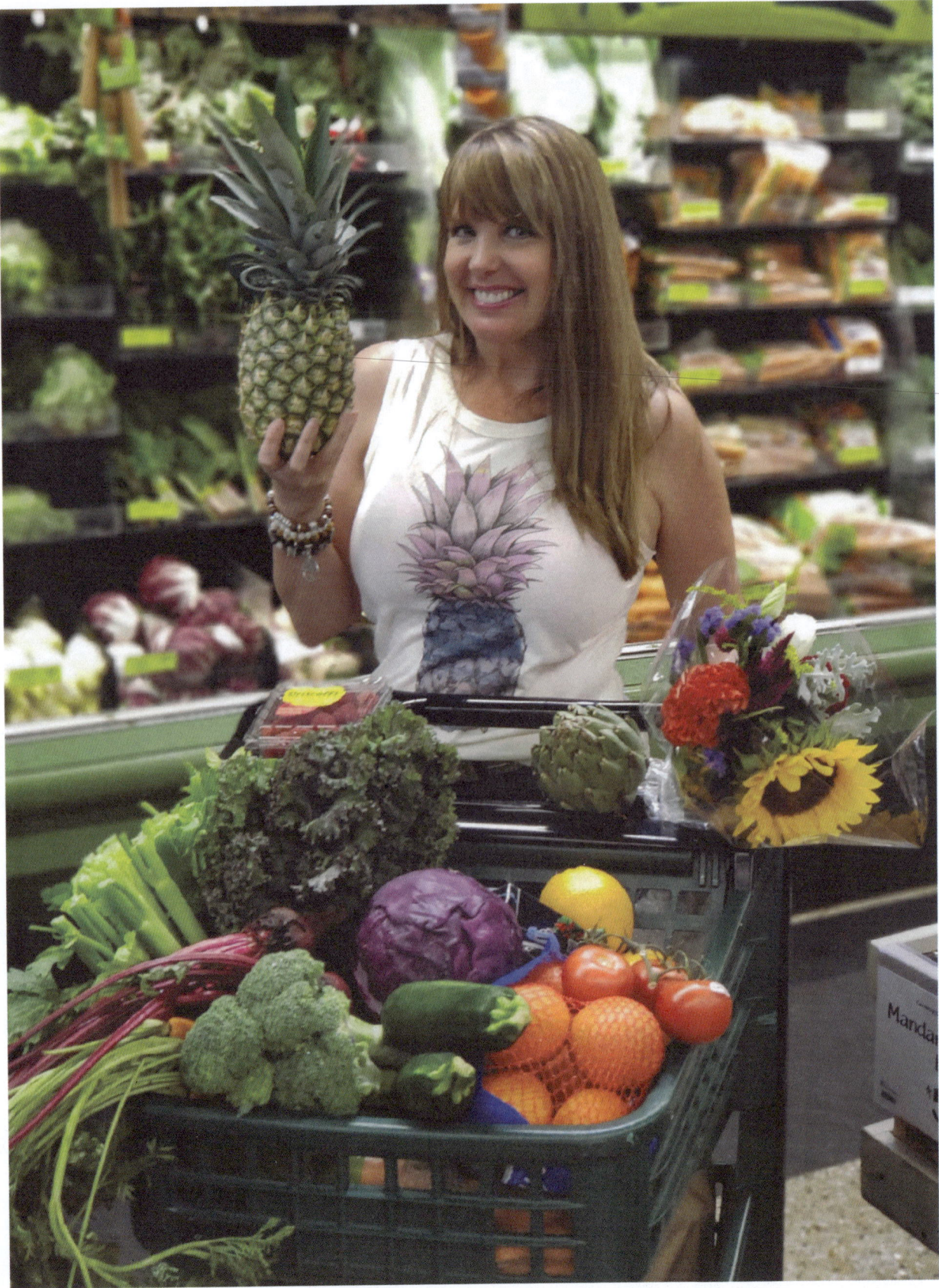

# Succeeding at your challenge

Have you ever felt alone in trying to live a healthier lifestyle and get into the habit of juicing? I've been there too, and I know how it feels.

So when I created this 30 day juicing challenge, I had a vision in mind. I imagined people of all ages not only juicing in their homes, but also spreading out and creating a sense of community. I saw people joining the challenge at work and having prizes for those who completed all 30 days. Spouses, partners, entire families brought closer together and living healthier lives because they decided to take the challenge together.

It's just one change. One habit that could change your life and take you in a new direction. So this is why I created the 30 day challenge, and I expect it to go further than my wild imagination has taken me so far.

Cheers to living your best life!

With much love,

*Tracee*

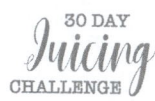

# From Visualization to Motivation

Sometimes remembering what a few of the vitamins and minerals do in the body can be very motivating!

**Vitamin C** helps to build cartilage, muscle, blood vessels and collagen in the bones. It aids in the absorption of iron, which is good for energy. Healthy eyesight and cardiovascular function are also benefits of vitamin C.

*Plant based sources of vitamin C:* kale, spinach, and other leafy greens. Kiwi, apples, oranges and other citrus fruits, berries, pineapple, tomatoes, broccoli and other cruciferous vegetables.

**Vitamin A** is a fat soluble vitamin, which means it is able to be stored inside of organs like the liver or in body fat. It is important for healthy vision and immune function. Vitamin A also helps the heart, lungs, kidneys, and other organs work properly.

*Plant based sources of vitamin A:* green leafy vegetables, broccoli, carrots, red bell peppers, sweet potatoes and squash. Cantaloupe, papaya, peaches, apricots, and mangoes.

**Vitamin K** is important for building and maintaining strong bones, normal blood clotting, and supporting heart health. This vitamin plays a role in normal bone metabolism and helps to generally ensure that calcium gets to the right places in the body, such as the bones and teeth.

*Plant based sources of Vitamin K:* leafy greens (kale, spinach, Swiss chard, turnip greens, mustard greens, parsley, and romaine lettuce), cruciferous vegetables (Brussels sprouts, broccoli, cabbage), asparagus, bok choy, parsley.

The body needs **calcium** to maintain and build strong teeth and bones. Calcium is also essential in carrying out many important functions such as contracting muscles, transmitting nerve signals, releasing hormones, and healthy blood clotting.

*Plant based sources of calcium:* kale, broccoli, collard greens, bok choy, watercress, mustard greens.

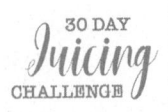

**Magnesium** is essential for synthesis of protein in the body, , nerve and muscle function, regulation of blood glucose and blood pressure. Roughly 60% of the magnesium in your body is found in bone, and the remainder is present in muscles, soft tissues and fluids. Every cell in the body contains magnesium it and needs it to function properly. Magnesium is extremely helpful for better exercise performance.

*Plant based sources of magnesium:* sea vegetables, dark leafy greens such as spinach and beet greens, tomatoes, lima beans, artichokes, and sweet potatoes.

**Potassium** is essential for normal, healthy function of all cells in the body. Not only does it regulate the heartbeat, but it also helps the muscles and nerves to function properly. Potassium is vital for carbohydrate and protein synthesis.

*Plant based sources of potassium:* watermelon, avocado, sweet potato, spinach, kale, medjool dates, bananas, beets, Swiss chard, oranges.

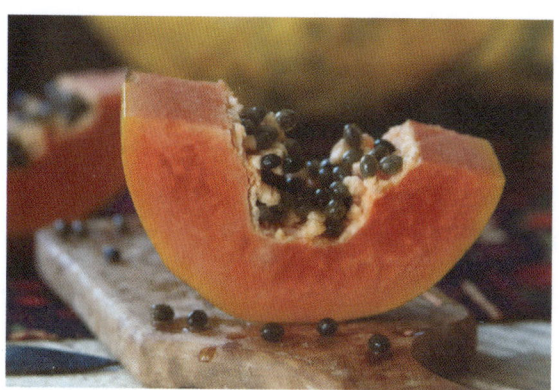
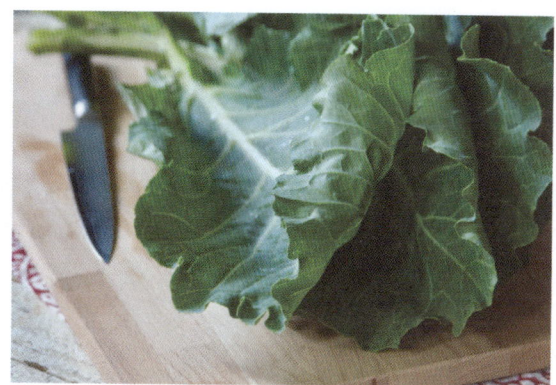

**Soluble fiber** is still in the juice when you remove the pulp with a juicer. This type of fiber attaches to cholesterol particles and removes them from the body, which can help lower LDL cholesterol. It also absorbs water and turns it into gel in the intestines, slowing digestion. Soluble fiber helps sugar to be absorbed more slowly and can help with blood glucose levels.

**Insoluble fiber** is the bulk fiber that is left in the pulp bin after you have finished juicing. This type of fiber helps food pass through the intestines more quickly and helps prevent constipation.

From Visualization to Motivation

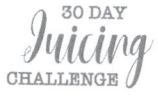

# Why Your Juicer Matters

Having the right juicer for you, your family and your lifestyle is vital. This decision can mean the difference between becoming a lifetime juicer or one who has joined the ranks of people who try it for a couple of weeks then banish their machine to the garage.

So often I see people buy the cheapest machine they can find, thinking they'll get a better one if they really enjoy it. This approach is similar to preparing a five-course meal using a butter knife to chop, peel, and slice the ingredients — inefficient, time consuming and discouraging.

**A juicer that works at a slow speed has many benefits:**

- Vital nutrients- vitamins, minerals and enzymes remain intact.
- Better tasting, higher quality and smoother texture of juice.
- Wheatgrass and leafy greens process more efficiently.
- Homemade almond milk can be made easily.
- Juice can be stored in the refrigerator for a longer period of time.
- Higher yield of juice and less waste.
- Pulp comes into the bin dry and finely processed.

Juice made with a high speed juicer begins to separate and turn brown almost immediately, and there is considerable waste. The pulp often contains chunks of cucumber and apple, while spinach and other greens come out almost whole in the pulp bin.

This is why I feel so passionate about having a good juicer! Over the years I've received so many letters from people who felt like they had failed, when really they may have succeeded at juicing if they had started with a good juicer. Juicing is an entirely different experience with the right tools!

The first time I did a side by side experiment, I was actually shocked at the results. After weighing the ingredients meticulously and making the same recipe in each juicer, the slow juicer produced an entire extra glass of brighter, tastier juice.

Although the investment of a quality juicer may seem significant at first, a good slow juicer will pay for itself in time, quality and yield of juice.

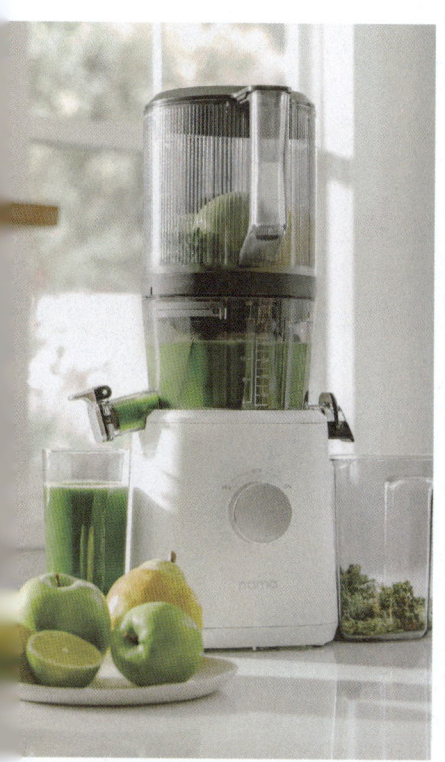
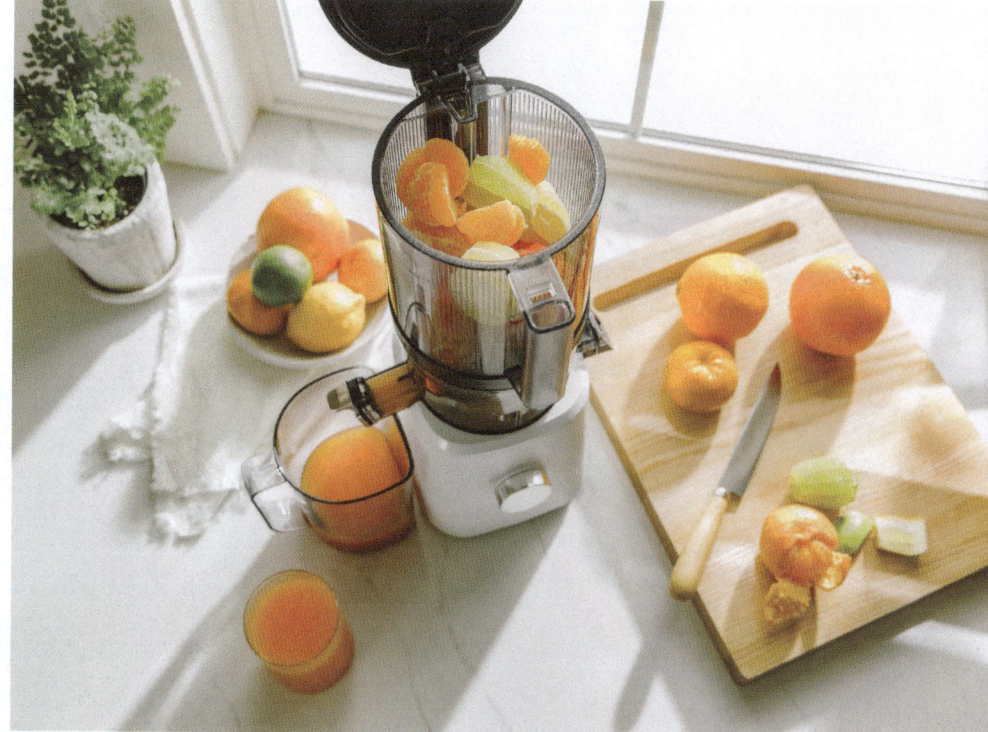

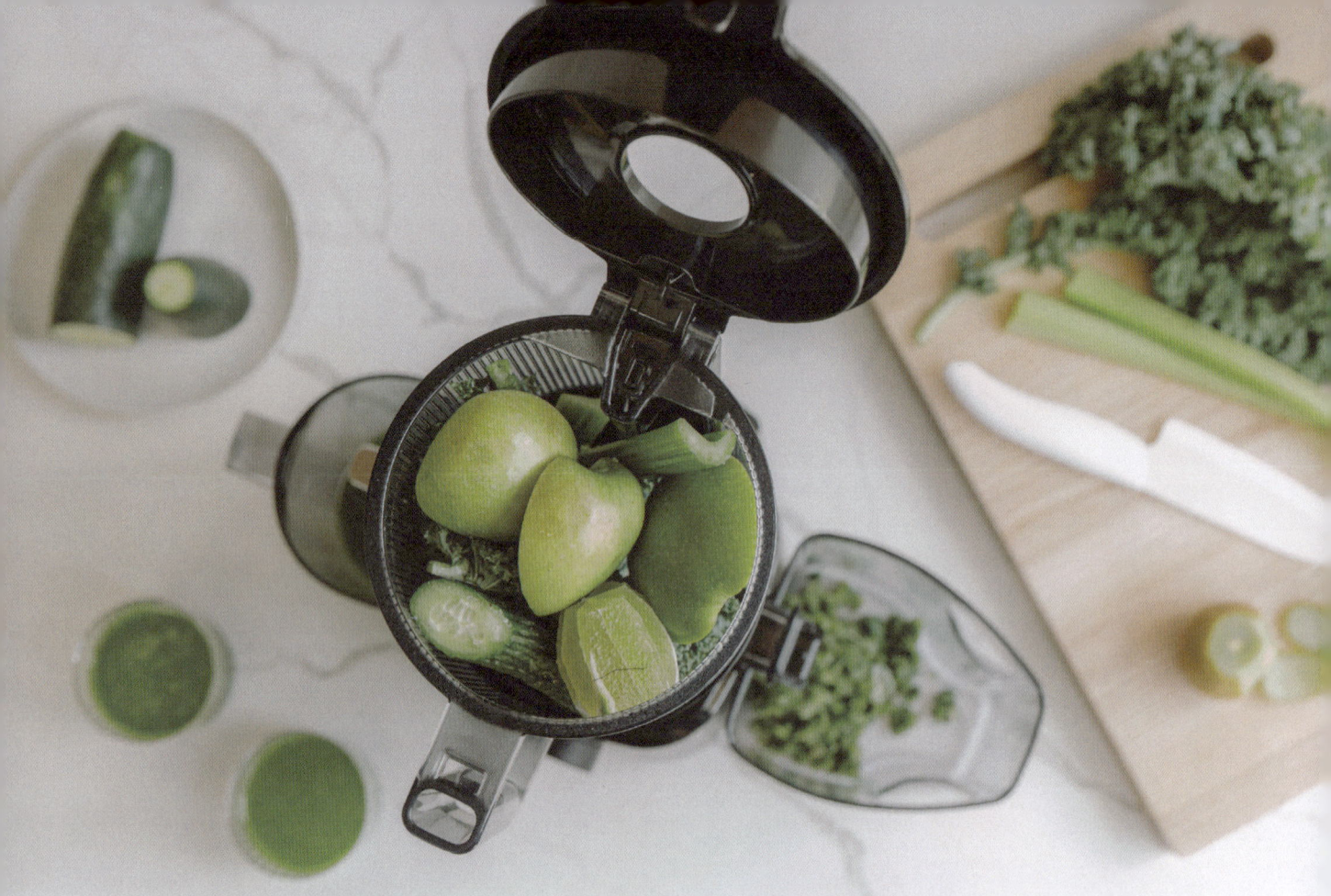

## My Favorite Juicer

Do you feel like having to chop and prep ingredients takes too much time? If so, you are not alone in feeling this way. I want you to know that you have been heard! For over three years, my friends at Nama have been working diligently to address your concerns and create a solution that will help you consume more plants and enjoy a healthier lifestyle.

The Nama J2 Cold Press Juicer has revolutionized juicing! Cutting and prep work are virtually a thing of the past. Fruits and vegetables are placed into the hopper without needing to be cut (except to remove large pits that could damage the juicer). **This new technology allows you to load an entire recipe at once, then step away.** On busy days, this hands free approach helps you to easily multitask while making your juice. Powerful yet quiet, this juicer can handle anything from leafy greens to soft fruits and hard root vegetables.

I am thoroughly impressed with the attention to detail that has gone into the Nama J2 itself. You can feel the quality of materials when you hold it in your hands. The parts are solid and made to last. The juicer is beautiful and fits easily under the kitchen cabinet while taking very little space on the counter. This is important to me, as I prefer to leave my juicer in plain view as part of my daily routine.

The juice this machine produces has a vibrant color and a smooth texture. The flavor is noticeably more appealing - an adventure for the tastebuds. This juicer works at a very slow speed, which allows vitamins, minerals and enzymes to remain intact.

The smoothie screen is another great feature. I use it to make my own homemade tomato sauce and salsa. The smoothie screen creates smoothies at a slow speed without needing to use a blender, preserving vital nutrients that can be lost at a high speed.

The almond milk the J2 produces has a wonderful flavor and a velvety texture. Many people have said this was the best almond milk they have ever had, with a much fresher taste than any they had purchased at a store.

Cleanup is also quick and easy. The juice can be stored for up to 72 hours — which saves time during busy weeks where it may not be possible to juice every day.

I have been dedicated to juicing for over 22 years, and nothing even comes close to this juicer. I am proud to recommend the Nama J2 Cold Press Juicer as my all time favorite juicing machine!

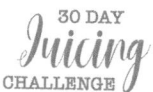

# Tips for Cleaning Your Juicer

Cleaning your juicer properly is important for both the function and beauty of the machine. Stains are much easier to prevent than to remove. Here are some time saving tips that will also help to keep your juicer running at peak performance.

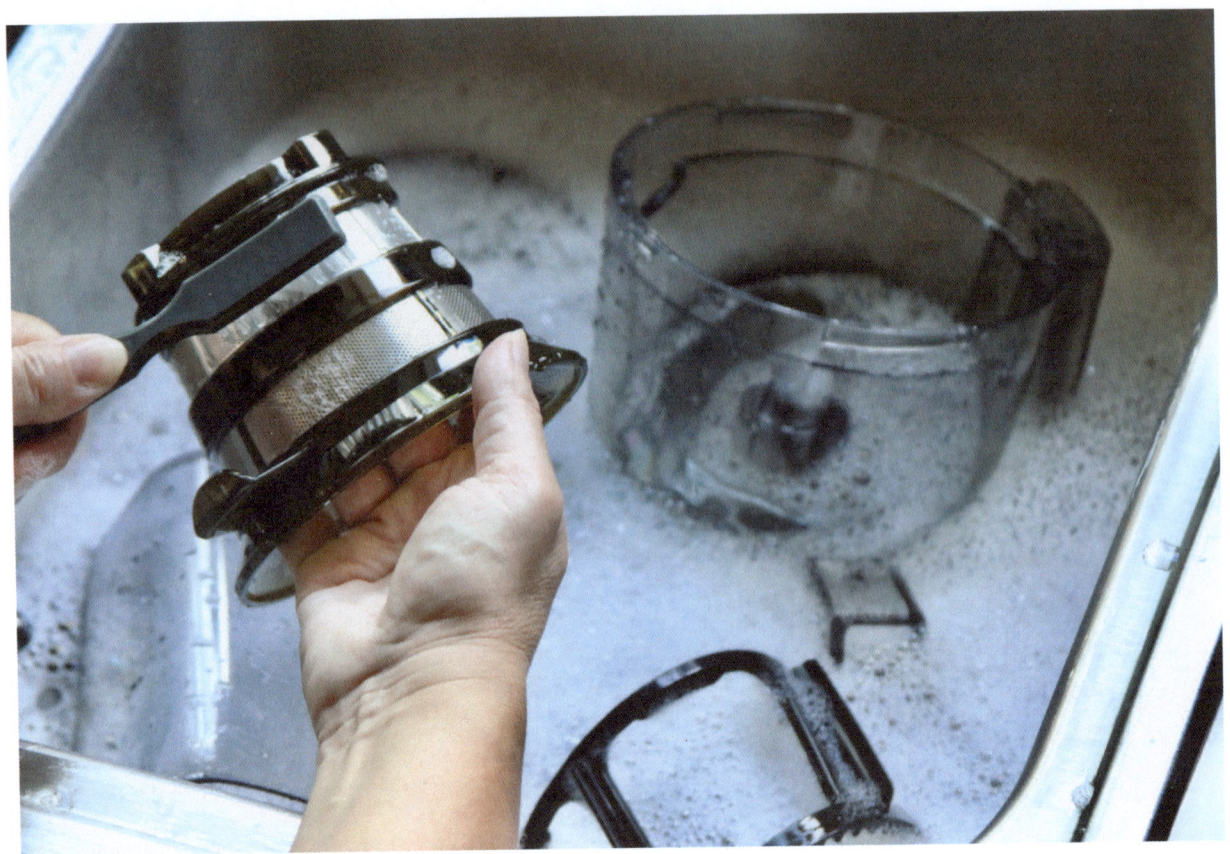

## Cleaning your juicer is so easy!

- Have a bowl of **hot, soapy water ready before you start to juice**, then put the juicer parts into it as soon as you finish juicing. This helps loosen the pulp inside of the parts and saves a little cleanup time.

- Keep your **juicing station fairly close to the sink**. The fewer steps you have to take, the faster the juicing and cleaning process will go.

- Adding **about 1/4 cup of peroxide to the soapy water** helps prevent stains and buildup that develops over time from carrots and other vegetables.

- **Using a brush to clean the screen** and not allowing pulp to build up on the screen helps with the yield of juice and performance of the juicer.

- **Cleaning your juicer right after juicing** makes the juicer much easier to clean. Although soaking it can help, washing the machine right after juicing saves time and helps prevent buildup and stains.

- Norwex EnviroCloths® are very helpful in **getting stains out of crevices** while using water alone to help remove stains and bacteria.

- **Using a soft cloth to immediately dry all of the juicer parts**, pitcher and pulp bin helps prevent water spots from forming on the equipment.

- **Lining the pulp bin** with a produce or grocery bag helps save time during cleaning.

- While trying to get more efficient at cleaning my juicer, I would set a timer and try to break my record. By **turning it into a game**, soon I was cleaning the machine in just a few minutes.

- Having a good slow juicer that is **fun to use and easy to clean** makes the cleaning less of a chore and more just a simple part of the juicing process.

# Tips for Storing Your Juice

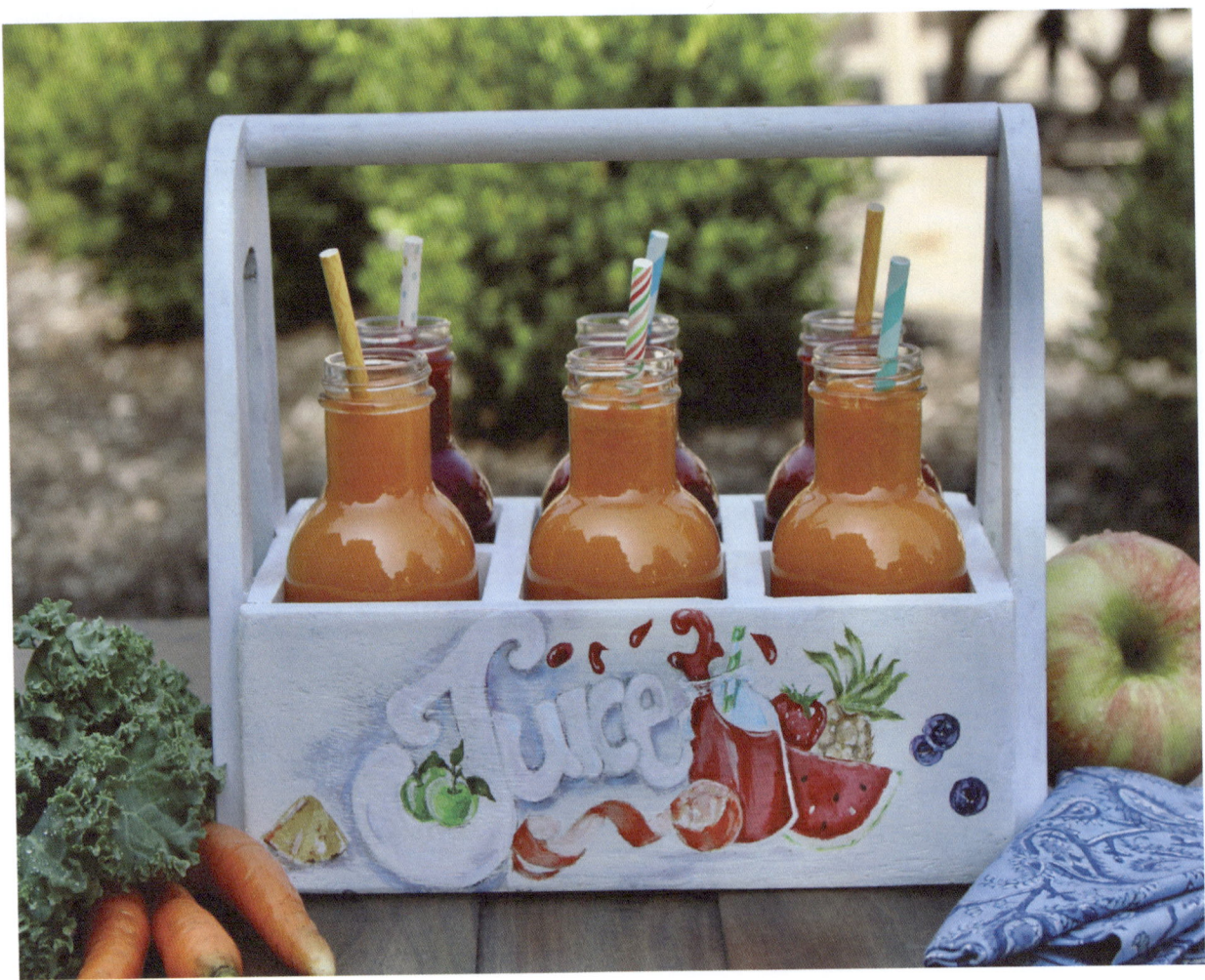

Although drinking juice immediately is preferred, storing juice ahead of time may be the most practical solution for your school or work schedule. Juice made with a twin gear, masticating, cold press, or other slow juicer may be stored for up to 72 hours. (I prefer to consume it within 24 to 48 hours.)

With a high-end centrifugal machine, you can usually store juice for up to 24 hours. However, many centrifugal machines require that you consume the juice immediately, as the high speed may cause the juice to oxidize quickly. For best results, check the owner's manual that comes with your juicing machine for maximum storage times.

How you store your juice is important for maximum shelf life:

- Use glass bottles or mason jars for fresh juice and nut milks.
- Store juice in the refrigerator immediately after preparing.
- Fill bottles or jars to the top leaving no air between the juice and the lid, to reduce exposure to oxygen.

When storing juice ahead of time, it is important to use fresh produce. Juicing fruits and vegetables to prevent them from spoiling is an excellent idea, but keep in mind that you may want to drink juice made with older produce sooner rather than later.

I add Himalayan salt to my fresh nut milks, not only for flavor and mineral content, but also to help the milk to last longer in the refrigerator.

Freezing your juice is also a storage option. I know a group of flight attendants who are gone for days at a time, and they have had great success with making their juice ahead of time and freezing it. BPA-free storage containers or bags work very well for storing juice in the freezer. Thaw juice in the refrigerator, then consume the juice immediately. (Frozen juice does have a slightly different texture when it thaws.)

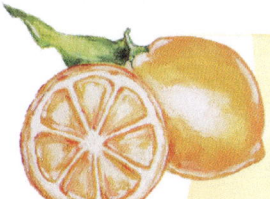

*Juicing a slice of lemon helps the juice maintain its vibrant color, especially when making ginger shots and fresh apple juice.*

Tips for Storing Your Juice 17

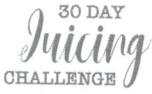

# Creating a Juicing Habit

Having a set time to make juice is one of the first steps in creating a new habit and having a successful challenge. If mornings are hectic, making juice in the evening for the next day may work better for you. Whatever you decide, making a commitment for 30 days and structuring life around that decision is key.

**Anchor juicing with an existing routine.** Say you make lunch in the evening for the next day. This may be a good time to make your juice for the following morning. If Saturday morning is dedicated to grocery shopping, this may be the ideal time to get your produce for your challenge also.

- After I make dinner, I will juice for tomorrow morning.
- After I take the kids to school, I will make today's recipe for the challenge.
- Before I do my Saturday grocery shopping, I will stop at the farmer's market and get what I can for this week's list.

**When the unexpected happens.** Perhaps some old friends came to town and invited you to dinner. By the time you get home, you just want to go to sleep. Knowing how long your routine takes and setting the alarm to juice first thing in the morning may be a workable alternate plan.

**Creating accountability.** Having a juicing partner or doing a group challenge can be powerful inspiration. Checking in at a set time each week or even a daily text or email is a small but effective step. Having a juice party and making the challenge recipes together is not only fun, but also creates a sense of community.

**Reward yourself!** Perhaps curling up with a book and drinking a glass of tea is something you don't get to enjoy very often. Creating an incentive that motivates you and indulging in it at the end of each week can add an element of fun to your challenge. This could be as simple as doing a 'happy dance' after drinking your juice each day.

**Visualize a successful, completed 30 days**. How will you feel at the end of 30 days if you juiced each day? Imagine that sense of accomplishment every day as though you have already completed it. See yourself as the person you have always wanted to become, doing the things you have always wanted to do. Just taking five minutes every morning and meditating in this way is another powerful tool for success. Keeping it visual keeps it vital.

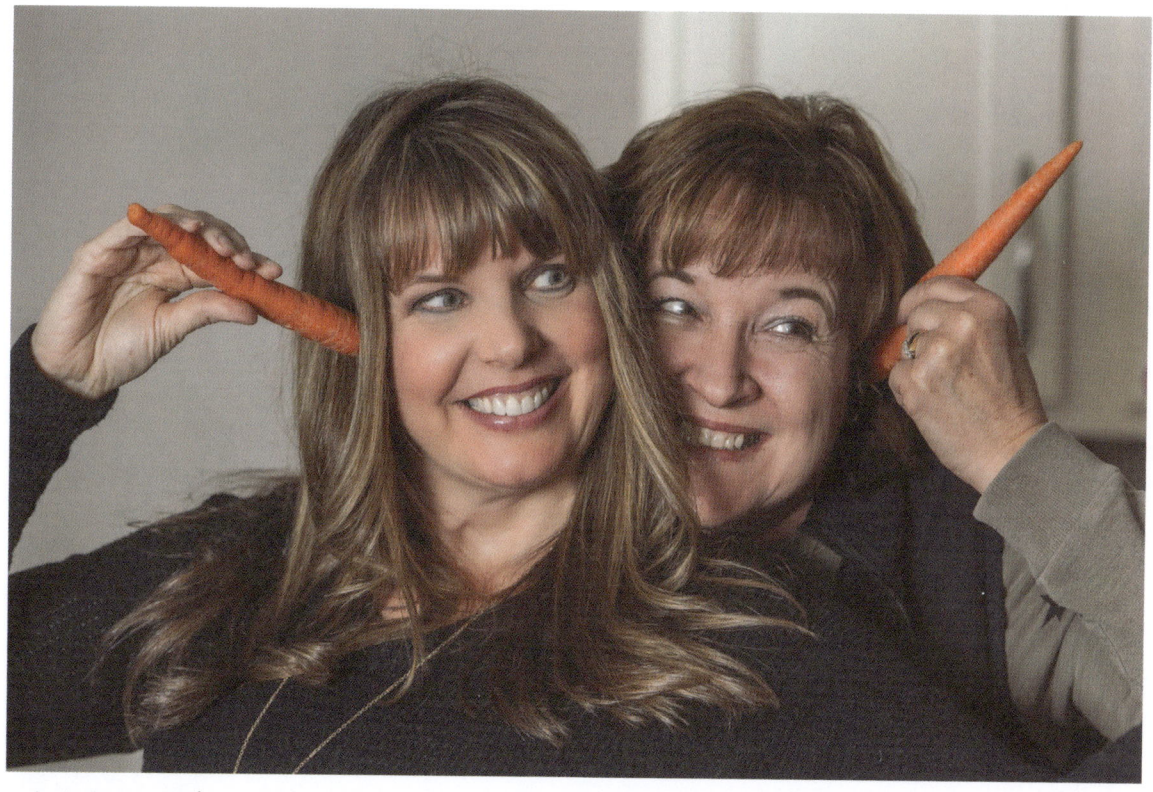

*Juicing with my Aunt Jackie in the kitchen. We got caught being silly.*

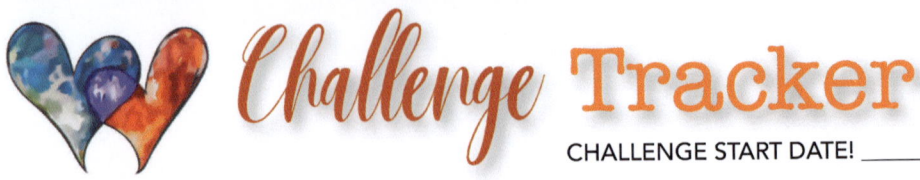

# Challenge Tracker

**CHALLENGE START DATE!** _____

| Day 1 | Day 2 | Day 3 | Day 4 | Day 5 |
|---|---|---|---|---|
| Liquid Sunshine ☐ | Green Detox ☐ | Turmeric Sunrise ☐ | Anytime Cocktail ☐ | The Eye Opener ☐ |

| Day 6 | Day 7 | Day 8 | Day 9 | Day 10 |
|---|---|---|---|---|
| Lemon Drop ☐ | Orchard Peach ☐ | Anytime Cocktail ☐ | Mean Green ☐ | Apple Crisp ☐ |

| Day 11 | Day 12 | Day 13 | Day 14 | Day 15 |
|---|---|---|---|---|
| Thai Green Magic ☐ | Orange Theory ☐ | Green Cheer ☐ | Heart Beet ☐ | Candy Crush ☐ |

| Day 16 | Day 17 | Day 18 | Day 19 | Day 20 |
|---|---|---|---|---|
| Green Ginger Ale ☐ | The Accelerator ☐ | Turmeric Sunrise ☐ | Cinnamint ☐ | Strawberry Mint Julep ☐ |

| Day 21 | Day 22 | Day 23 | Day 24 | Day 25 |
|---|---|---|---|---|
| The Eye Opener ☐ | Sweet Adeline ☐ | Fennelicious ☐ | Lemon Drop ☐ | Green Power ☐ |

| Day 26 | Day 27 | Day 28 | Day 29 | Day 30 |
|---|---|---|---|---|
| First Love ☐ | Power Aid ☐ | The Game Changer ☐ | Dr. Oz's Green Drink ☐ | Candy Crush ☐ |

# Tracking Your Progress

Studies have shown that joy, fulfillment and an overall sense of well being can result when personal goals are met. One powerful yet simple way to reach those goals is by tracking daily progress. Preparing and drinking one juice a day is a big deal!

The challenge tracker was created as a tool to stay motivated and to keep your challenge visual. Printing your challenge and having it in a place where it is seen every day can be very helpful.

**Keeping it visual keeps it vital!**

Each recipe is filled out for you in the tracker, and there is a blank square on the bottom right for you to check the box after you have completed that day's recipe.

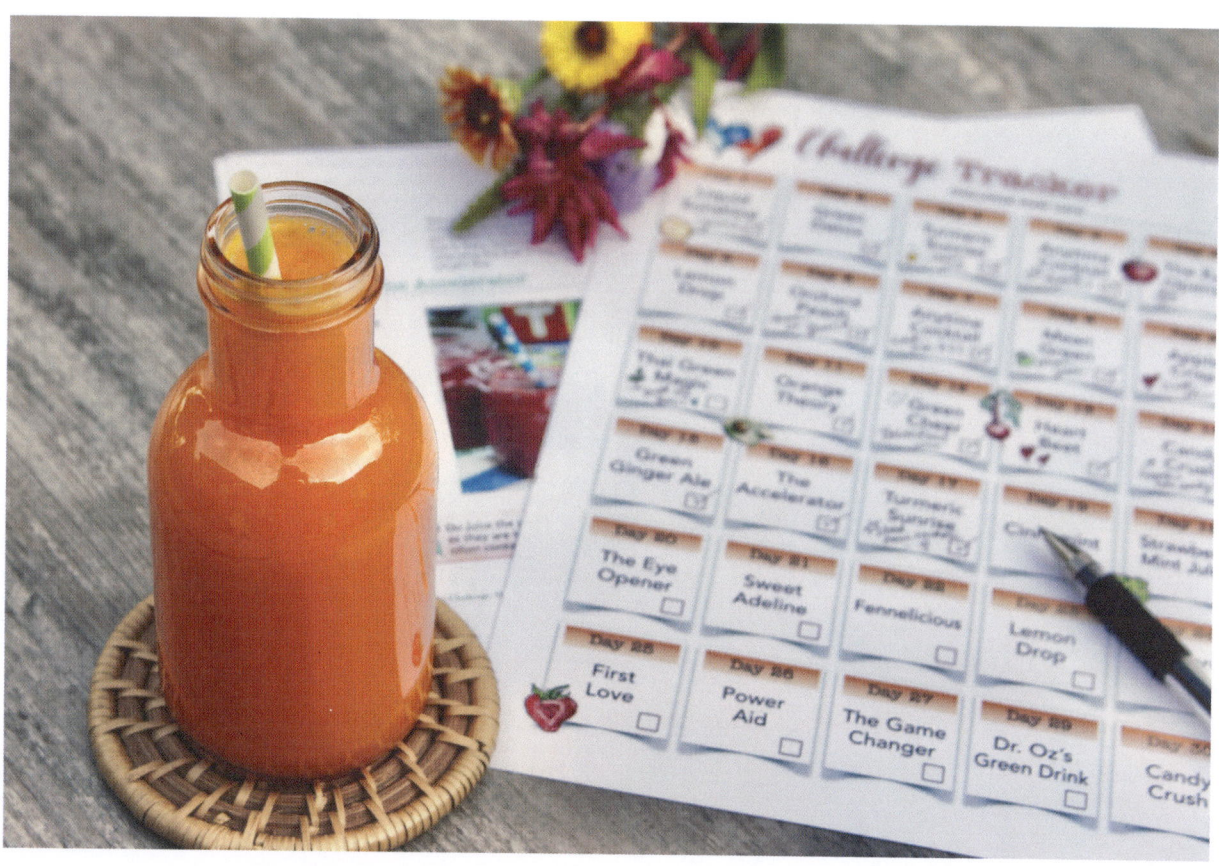

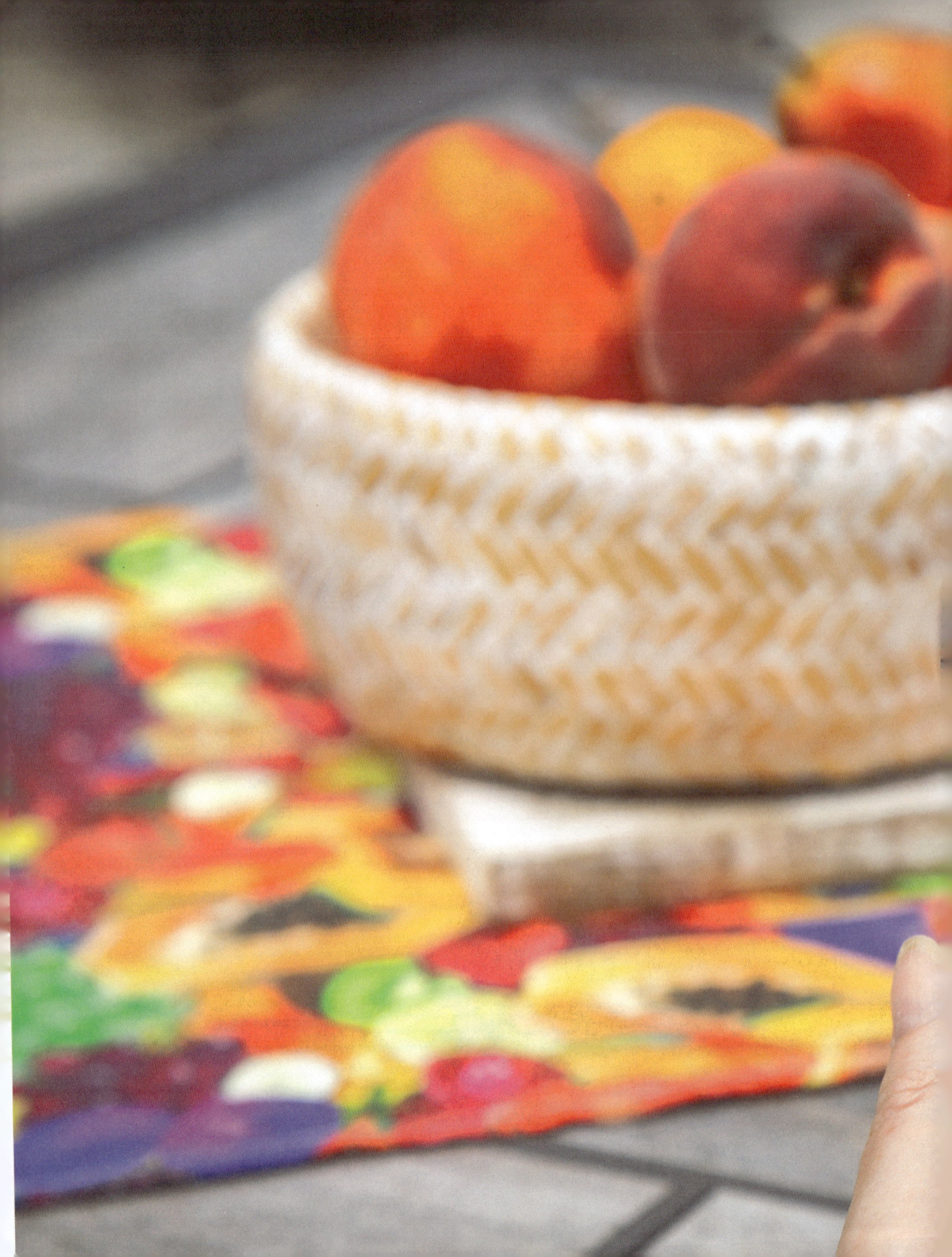

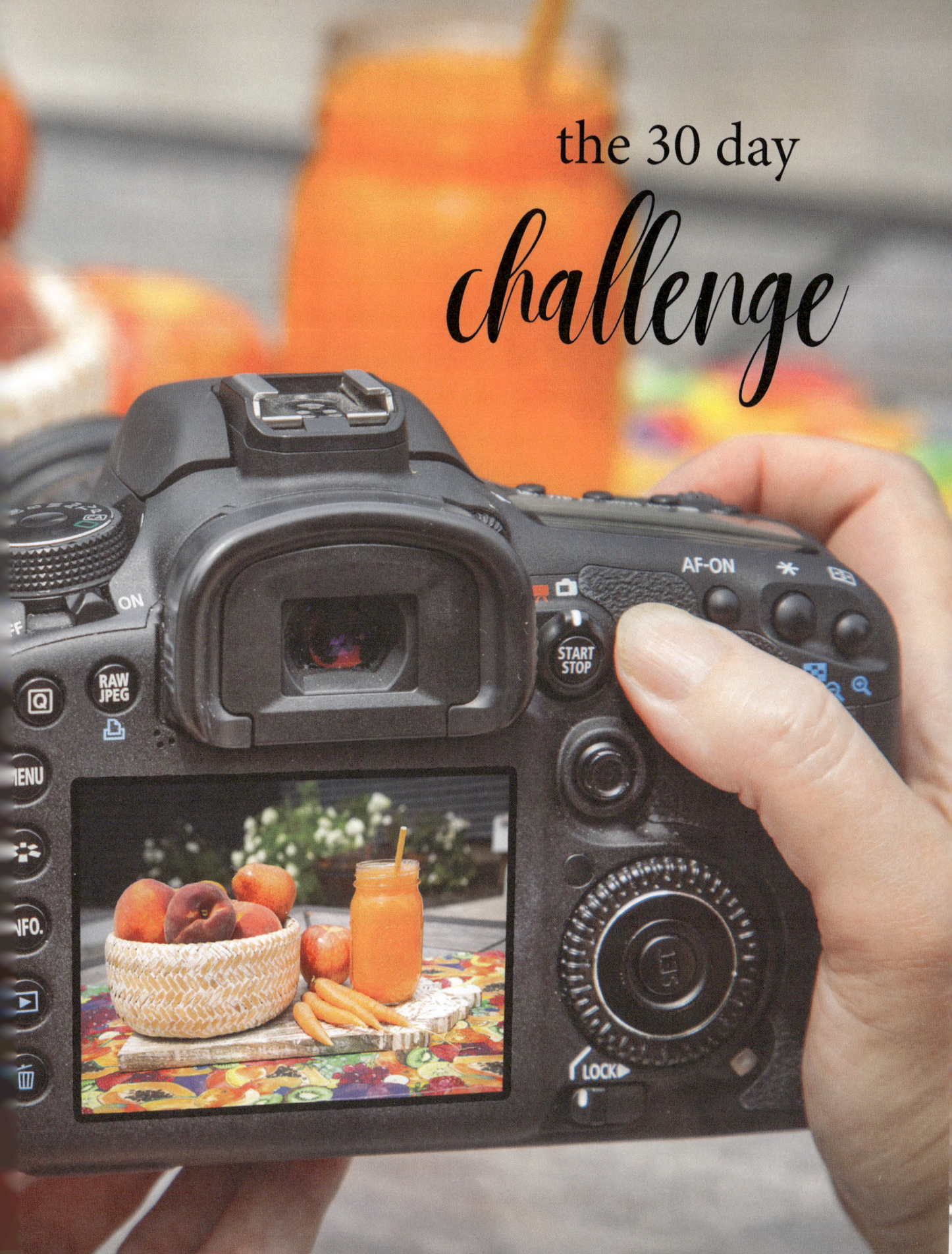

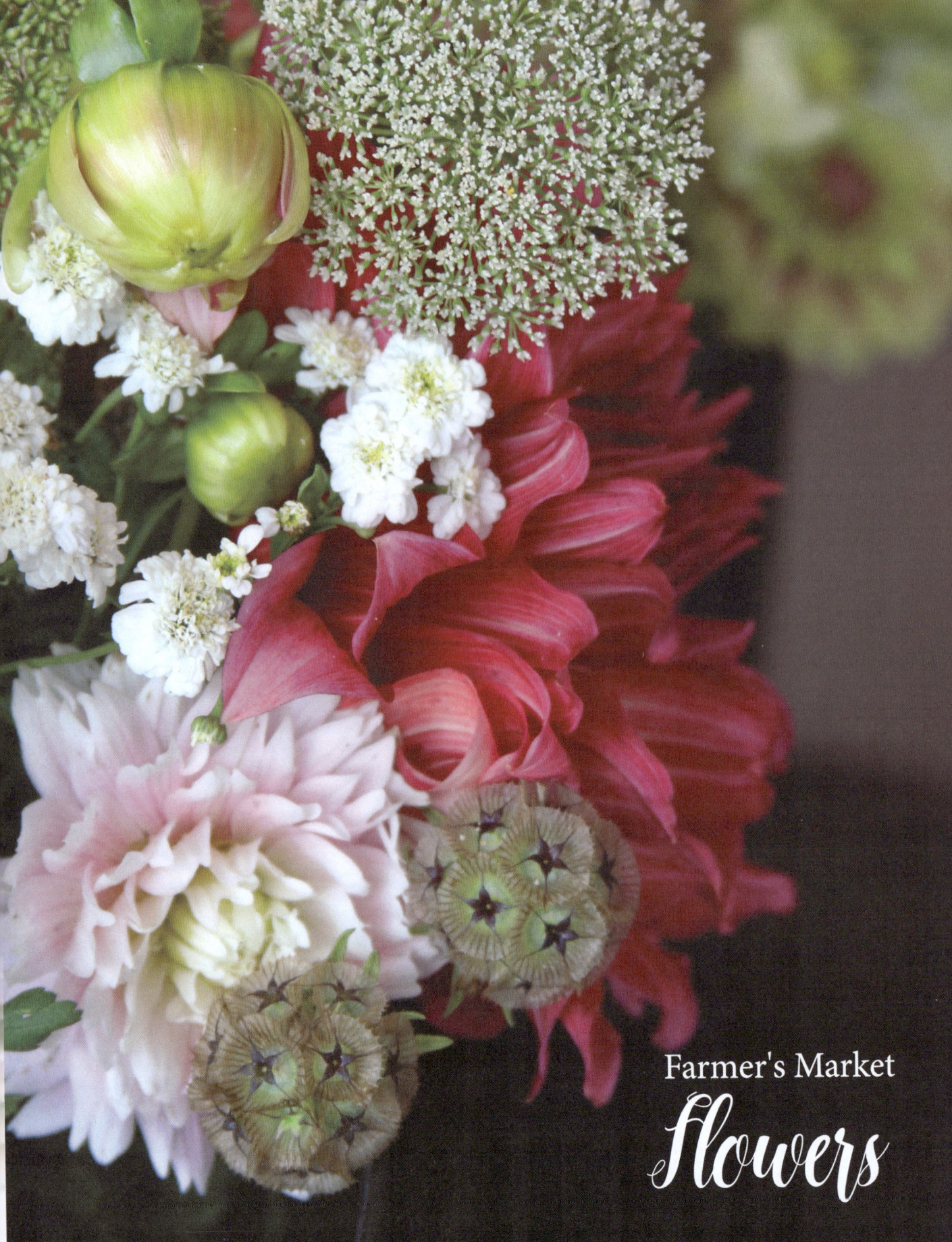

Farmer's Market *Flowers*

# Days 1-7 Shopping List

**Orange Week!** Having a list of ingredients saves time and money by eliminating multiple trips to the store and avoiding waste. Use this handy list to make your first seven days of juicing easy and fun!

## Vegetables

- [ ] 37 carrots
- [ ] 15 pieces celery
- [ ] 2 cucumbers
- [ ] 5 kale leaves
- [ ] 1 sweet potato
- [ ] 1 zucchini

## Fruits

- [ ] 14 apples
- [ ] 5 lemons
- [ ] 1 lime
- [ ] 7 oranges
- [ ] 2 peaches
- [ ] 4 pears

## Herbs & Spices

- [ ] 1 bunch parsley
- [ ] 6 inches ginger
- [ ] 6 inches turmeric

Just a reminder that the 30 day challenge is not a cleanse, but rather 30 days of recipes designed to help incorporate juicing into daily life.

Each recipe makes about 32 ounces of juice — enough for two people to have one 16-ounce glass each, per day, while still having solid food.

I have juice at different times, but I prefer to have recipes with more fruit earlier in the day.

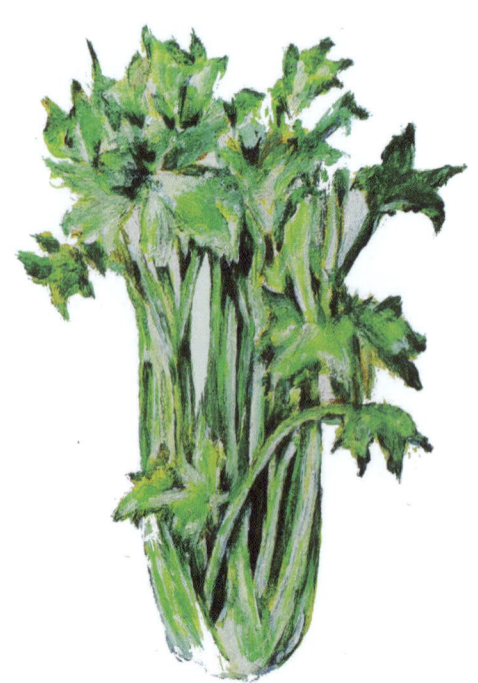

# DAY 1
## Liquid Sunshine

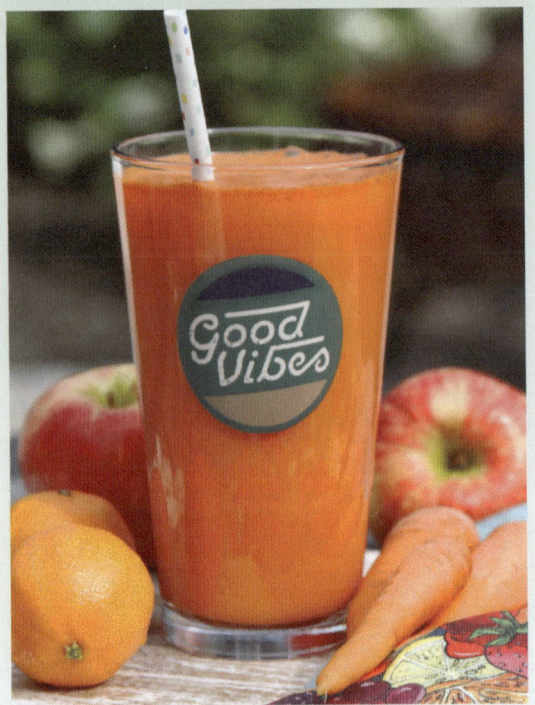

### Ingredients
- 2 apples
- 6 carrots
- 1 orange, peeled
- 1 sweet potato
- 1 inch ginger
- 1/2 lemon
- 2 celery

*Yield: 30 ounces*

# DAY 2
## Green Detox

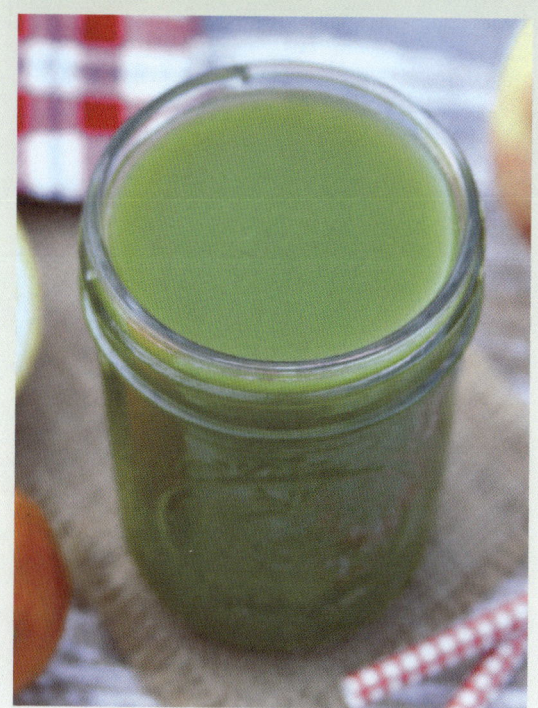

**Ingredients**

- 8 pieces celery
- 2 apples
- 1 orange, peeled
- 1 lime
- 1 cucumber
- 2 inches ginger

*Yield: 35 ounces*

# DAY 3
## Turmeric Sunrise

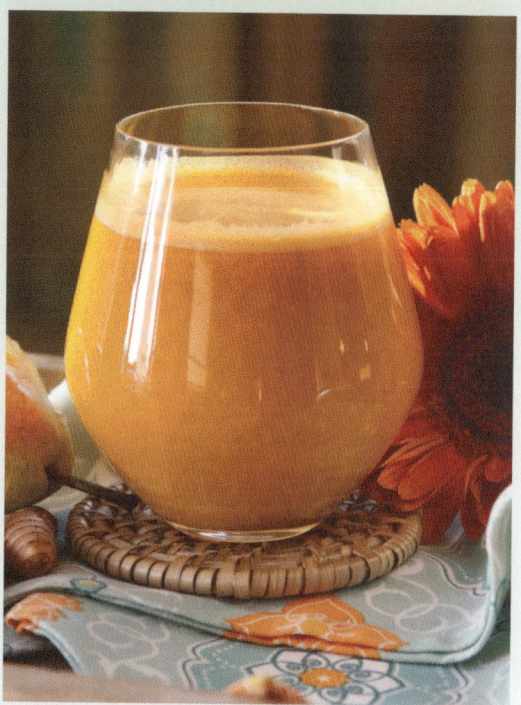

**Ingredients**

- 2 apples
- 3 carrots
- 3 celery
- 1 inch ginger
- 2 lemons, peeled
- 2 pears
- 6 inches turmeric (or 1 teaspoon powdered)

*Yield: 30 ounces*

# DAY 4
## The Anytime Cocktail

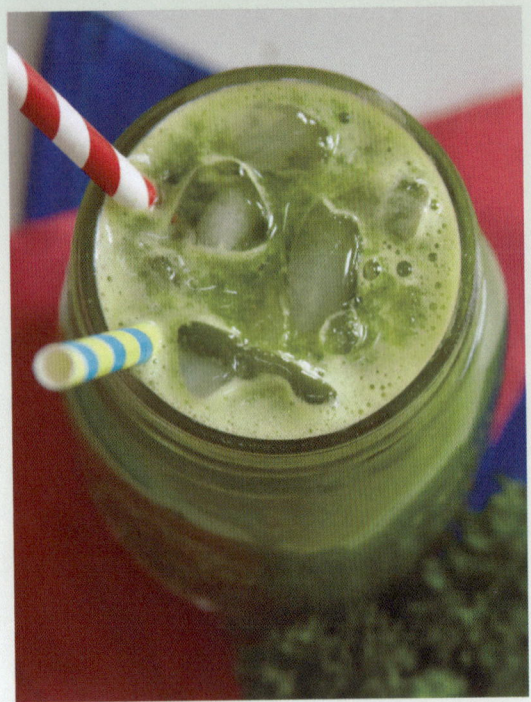

### Ingredients
- 2 apples
- 2 pieces celery
- 1 cucumber
- 5 kale leaves
- 1/2 lemon
- 2 oranges, peeled
- 1 handful parsley

Yield: 30 ounces

# DAY 5
## The Eye Opener

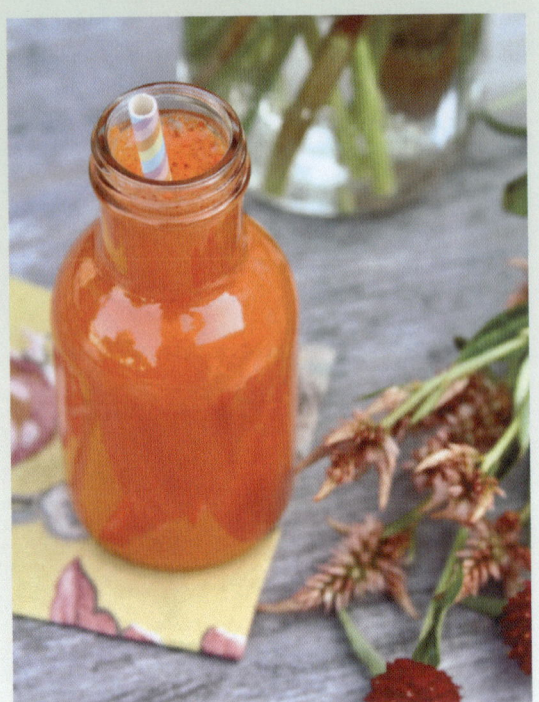

### Ingredients
- 2 apples
- 14 carrots
- 2 oranges, peeled

Yield: 30 ounces

# DAY 6

## Lemon Drop

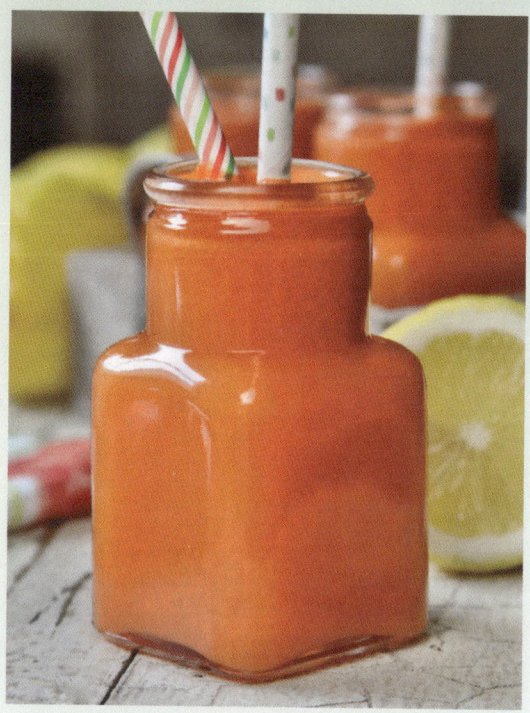

### Ingredients

- 2 apples
- 4 carrots
- 2 inches ginger
- 1 lemon, peeled
- 2 pears
- 1 zucchini

*Yield: 32 ounces*

# DAY 7

## Orchard Peach

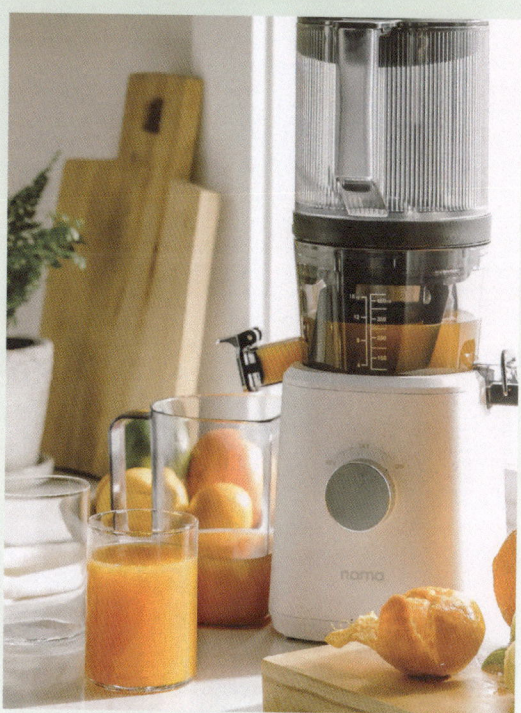

### Ingredients

- 2 apples
- 10 carrots
- 1/2 lemon
- 1 orange, peeled
- 2 large peaches

*Yield: 32 ounces*

*Yield*
30 ounces

Carrots and carrot juice boost the immune system by helping to protect the body against damage from free radicals, harmful bacteria, inflammation and viruses. Lemons help increase iron absorption, flush out the kidneys and improve the skin.

# Day 1: Liquid Sunshine

## Ingredients

- 2 apples
- 6 carrots
- 1 orange, peeled
- 1 sweet potato
- 1 inch ginger
- 1/2 lemon
- 2 celery

"Whatever good things we build end up building us."

— Jim Rohn

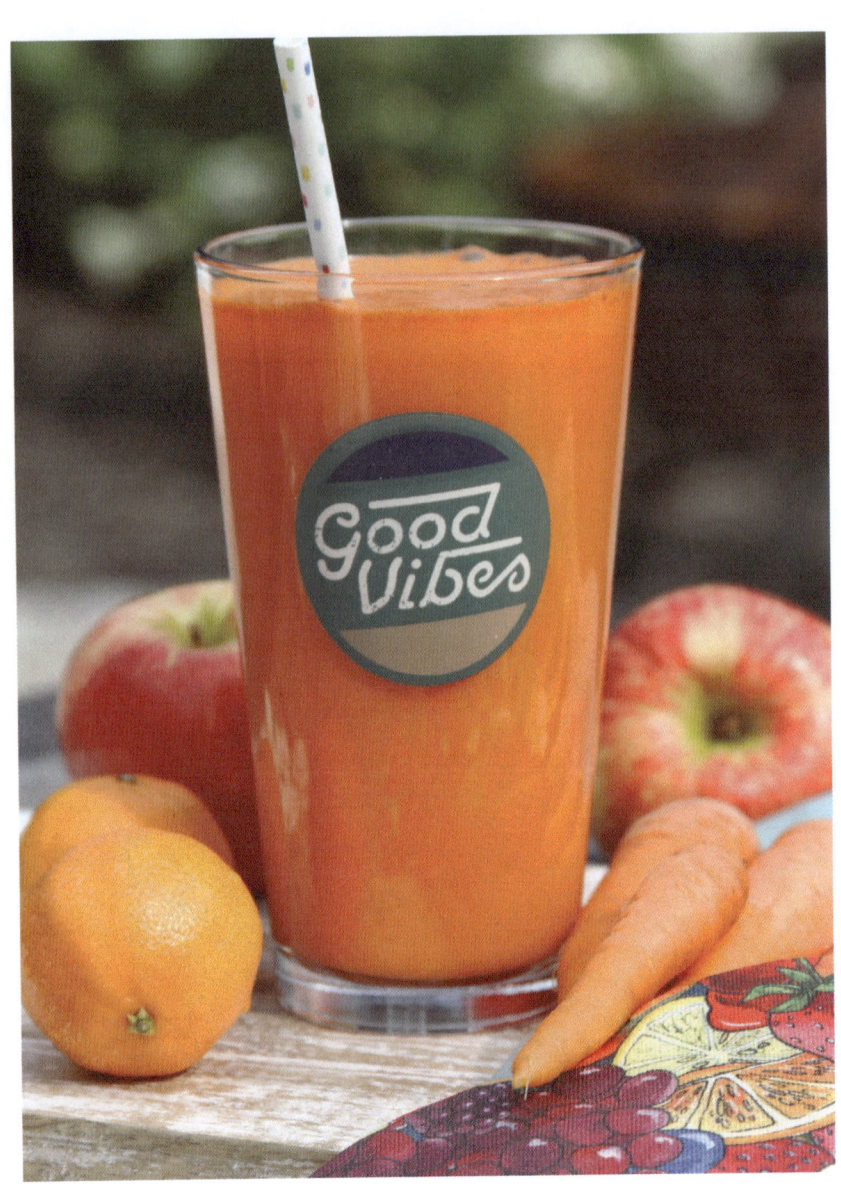

## Yield
35 ounces

This recipe has been very helpful as a transitional juice for those who want to drink celery juice but need other ingredients to get used to the taste.

# Day 2: Green Detox

## Ingredients

- 8 pieces celery
- 2 apples
- 1 orange, peeled
- 1 lime
- 1 cucumber
- 2 inches ginger

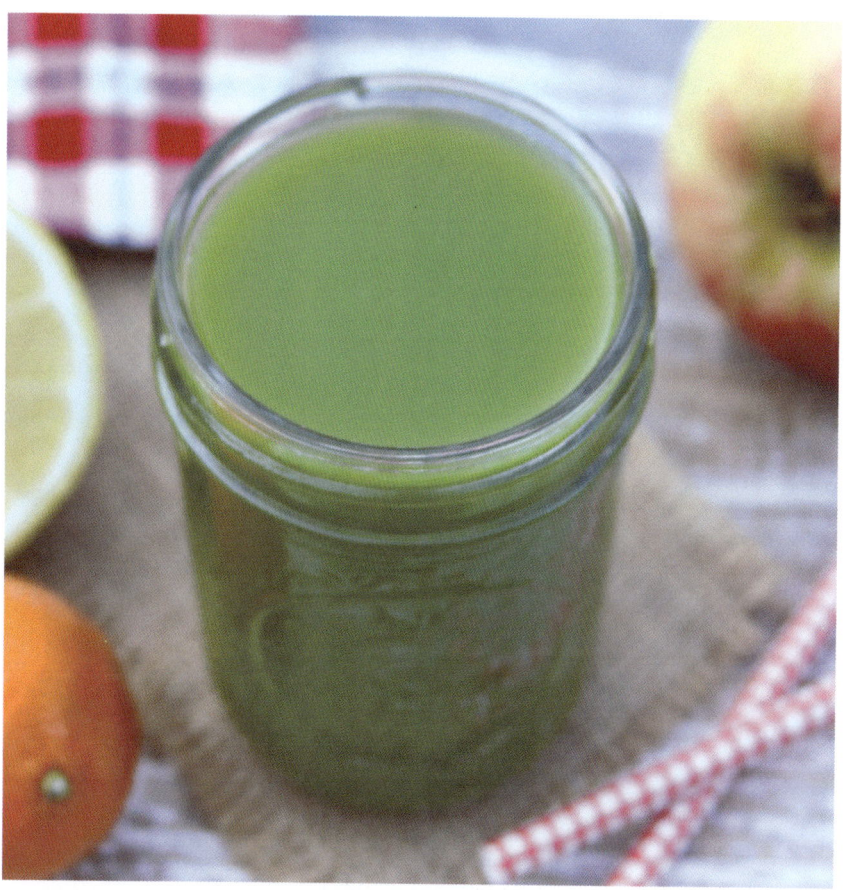

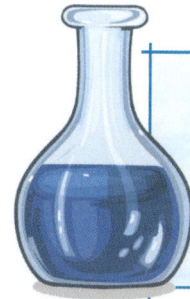

Studies have shown celery to be effective in reducing dangerous fat buildup in the liver and improvement in liver enzyme function.

Yield
30 ounces

I add freshly cracked pepper to this recipe. Studies have shown that combining black pepper with turmeric increases its absorption in the body by up to 2,000 percent.

# Day 3: Turmeric Sunrise

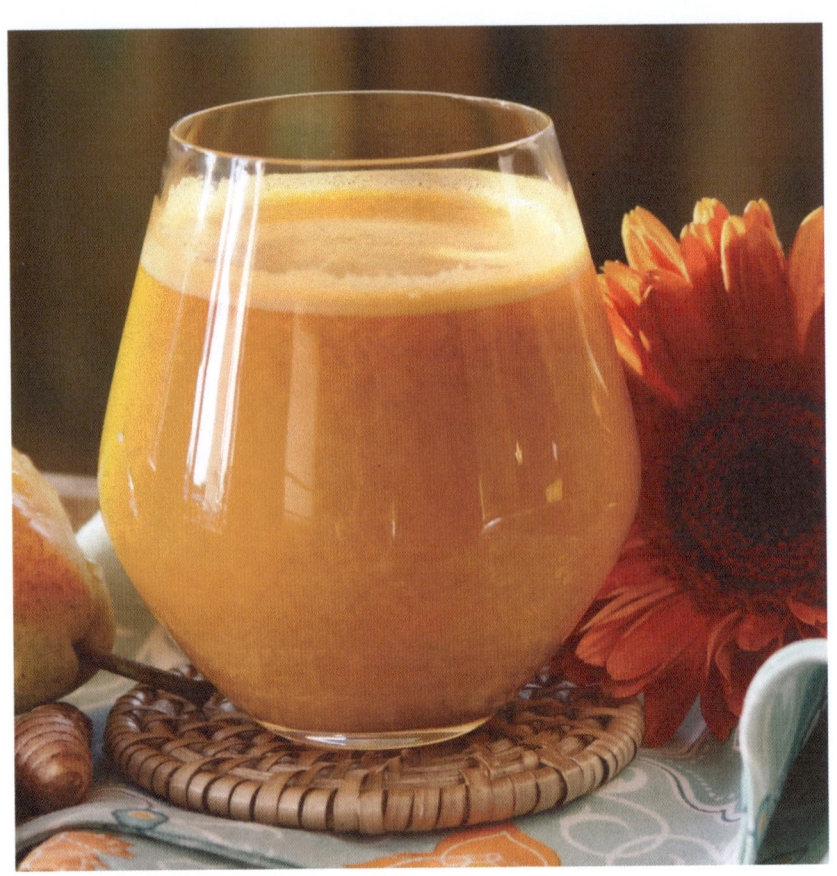

## Ingredients

- 2 apples
- 3 carrots
- 3 celery
- 1 inch ginger
- 2 lemons, peeled
- 2 pears
- 6 inches turmeric (or 1 teaspoon powdered)

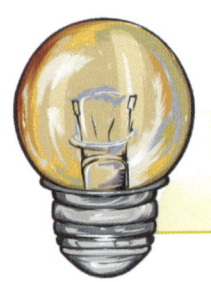

*If you don't have fresh turmeric, you can substitute with 1 teaspoon of powdered.*

*Yield*
30 ounces

Lemon is a natural diuretic, helping remove excess water weight from the body. Lemon and parsley combined are excellent kidney cleansers.

# Day 4: The Anytime Cocktail

## Ingredients

- 2 apples
- 2 pieces celery
- 1 cucumber
- 5 kale leaves
- 1/2 lemon
- 2 oranges, peeled
- 1 handful parsley

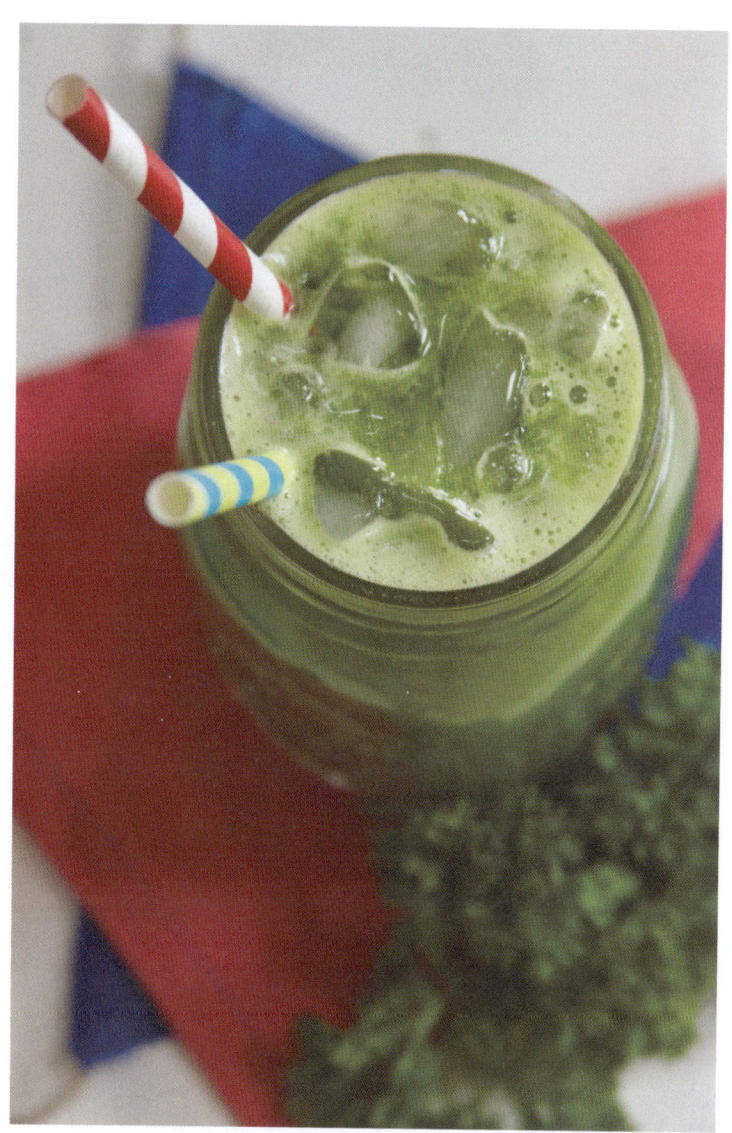

"The best thing about the future is that it comes one day at a time."

— Abraham Lincoln

**Yield**
30 ounces

*This is a perfect beginner recipe, as it contains only three ingredients, is easy to make, and it tastes delicious.*

# Day 5: The Eye Opener

## Ingredients

- 2 apples
- 14 carrots
- 2 oranges, peeled

"The smallest of disciplines, practiced every day, start an incredible process that can change our lives forever."

— Jim Rohn

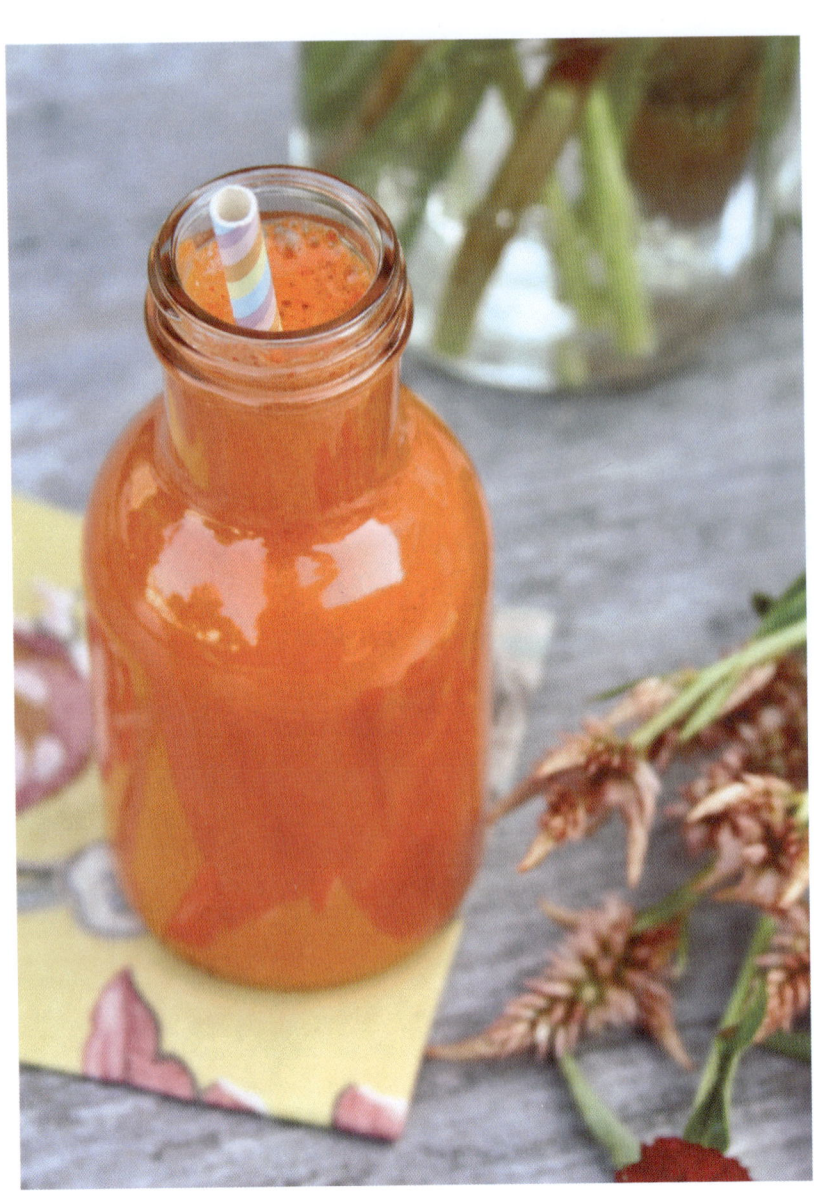

## Yield
32 ounces

*Pears are high in Vitamin C and antioxidants. They are good for the heart and may help with weight loss.*

# Day 6: Lemon Drop

### Ingredients
- 2 apples
- 4 carrots
- 2 inches ginger
- 1 lemon, peeled
- 2 pears
- 1 zucchini

*"A little progress each day adds up to big results."*

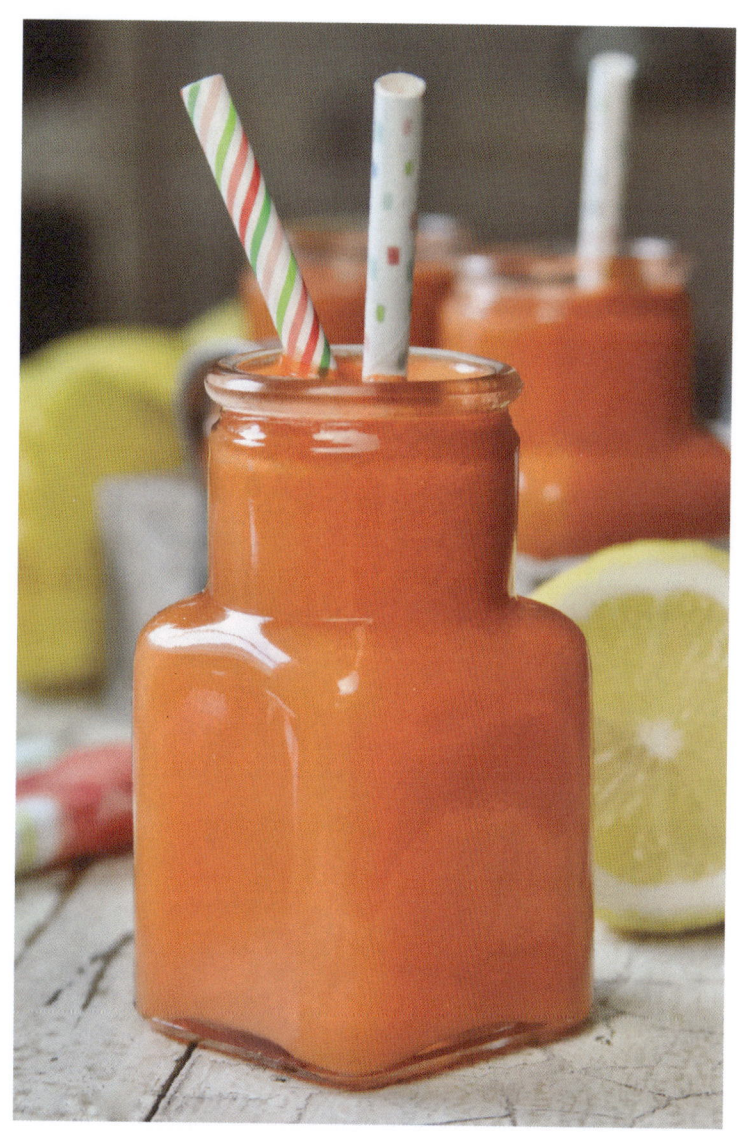

The Challenge: Days 1-7   35

## Yield
32 ounces

*If peaches are not in season in your area, you can use 1 cup of frozen peaches, adding them in between the fresh produce. Juicing frozen fruit all at once will produce a sorbet rather than juice.*

# Day 7: Orchard Peach

## Ingredients

- 2 apples
- 10 carrots
- 1/2 lemon,
- 1 orange, peeled
- 2 large peaches

"All our dreams can come true if we have the courage to pursue them."

— Walt Disney

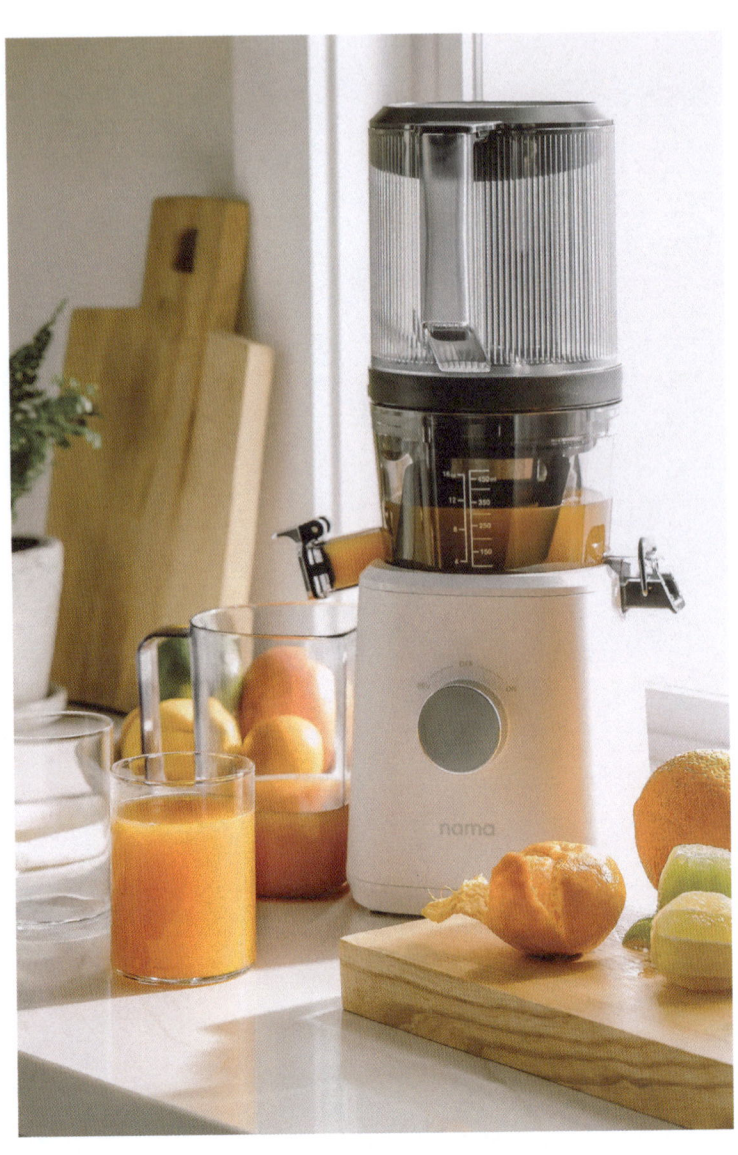

# Days 1-7 Assessment

What were my strongest points this week?

_____

_____

_____

Did I juice or have juice every day of the challenge?_____

What was my favorite recipe? _____

Were there any unexpected obstacles? If so, how did I handle them with regards to juicing?

_____

_____

_____

Is there anything I can do to prepare for next week to make it even better?

_____

_____

_____

Farmer's Market
*radishes*

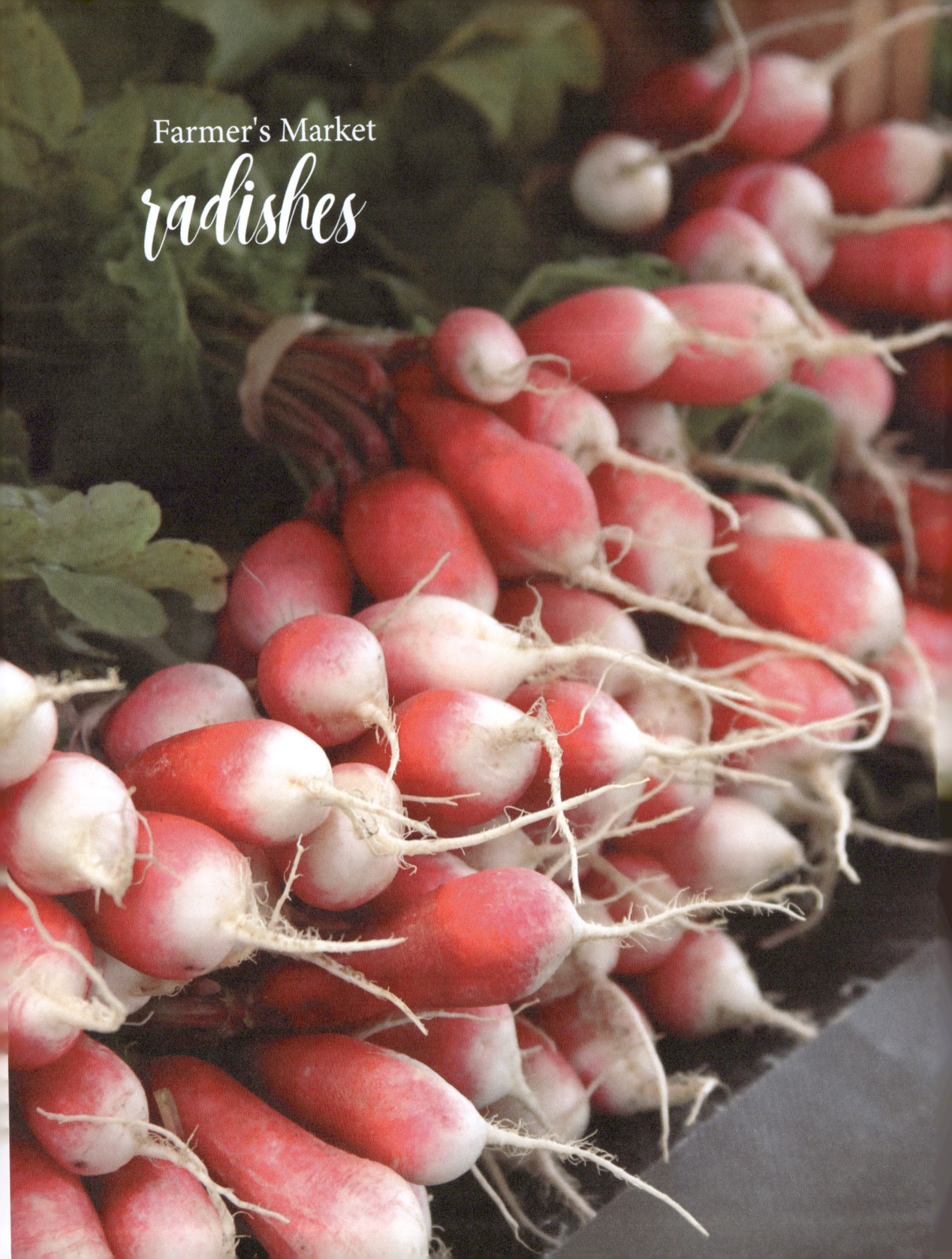

# Days 8-14 Shopping List

**Green Week!** This second week contains recipes that have more leafy greens, celery and spinach. Hope you have scheduled a time for shopping and have created a routine that works best for you.

## Vegetables
- [ ] 1 avocado
- [ ] 1 beet
- [ ] 12 carrots
- [ ] 12 pieces celery
- [ ] 4 cucumbers
- [ ] 11 kale leaves
- [ ] 5 cups spinach
- [ ] 2 sweet potatoes

## Fruits
- [ ] 16 apples
- [ ] 1 cup grapes
- [ ] 3 lemons
- [ ] 10 oranges

## Herbs & Spices
- [ ] cinnamon
- [ ] 12 Thai basil leaves
- [ ] 4 inches ginger
- [ ] 1 bunch curly parsley
- [ ] 1 bunch Italian parsley

As you begin week two, are you looking forward to your next juice? Whether juicing by yourself or with a partner, may you feel so motivated that you lead the way and inspire others to stay on track with their own personal goals.

Each recipe this week also makes about 32 ounces of juice — enough for two people to have one 16-ounce glass each, per day, while still having solid food. If you have a partner who wants to join you, it's not too late!

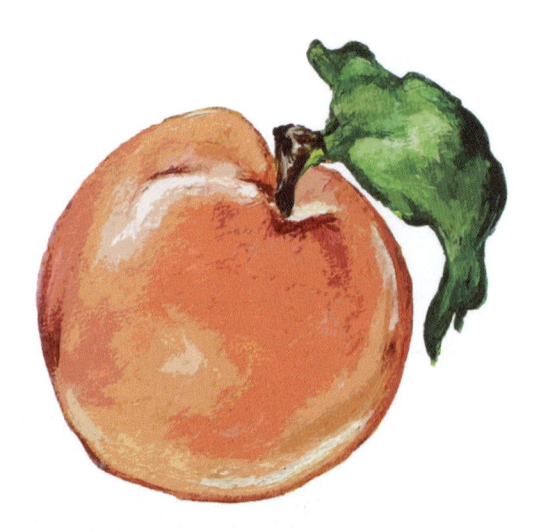

# DAY 8

## The Anytime Cocktail

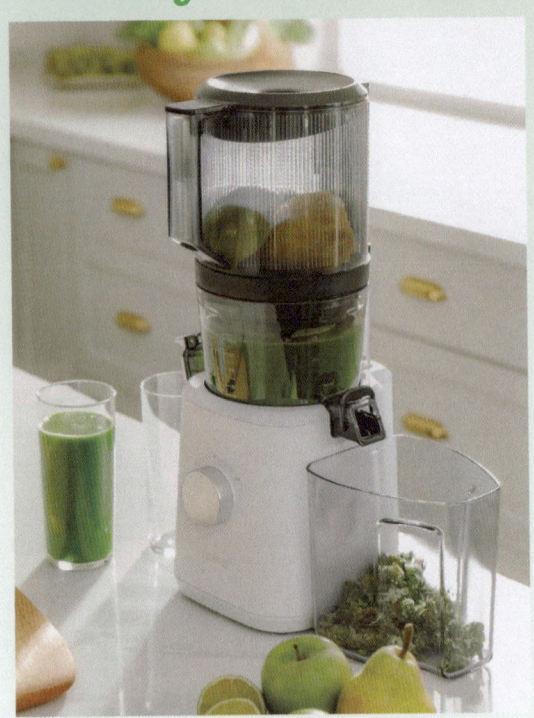

### Ingredients

- 2 apples
- 2 celery
- 1 cucumber
- 5 kale leaves
- 1/2 lemon
- 2 large oranges, peeled
- 1 handful parsley

Yield: 30 ounces

# DAY 9
## Mean Green

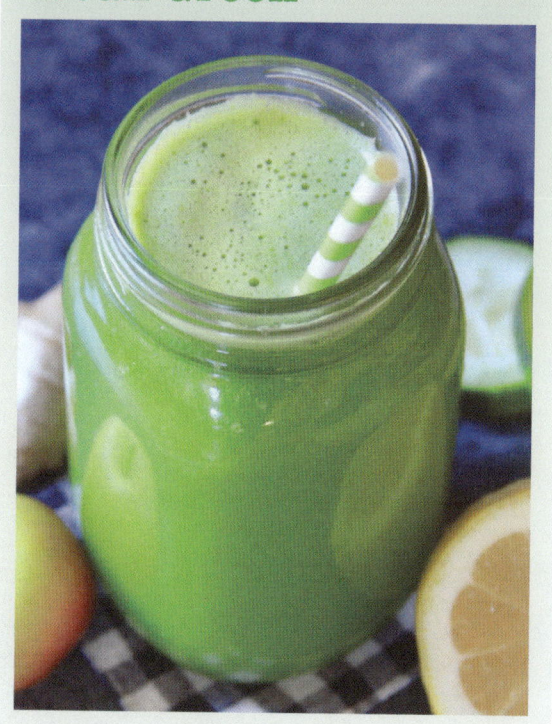

### Ingredients
- 2 apples
- 4 celery
- 1 cucumber
- 1 inch ginger
- 6 kale leaves
- 1/2 lemon

*Yield: 32 ounces*

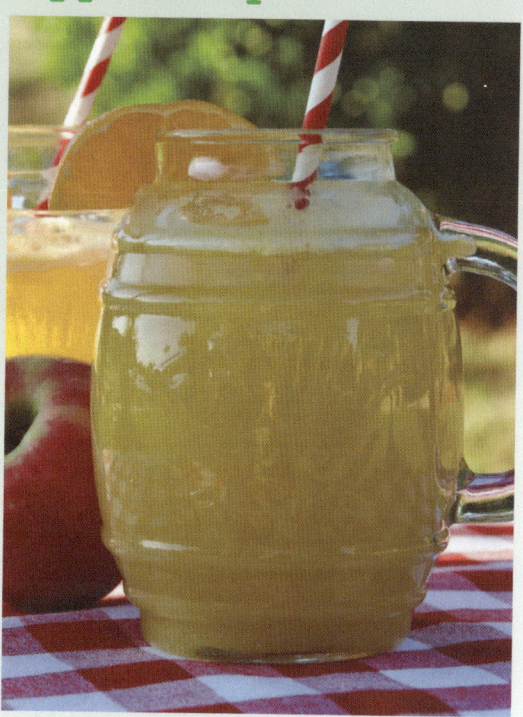

# DAY 10
## Apple Crisp

### Ingredients
- 5 apples
- 2 oranges, peeled
- 2 celery

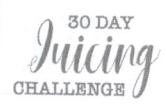

*Yield: 30 ounces*

# DAY 11

## Thai Green Magic

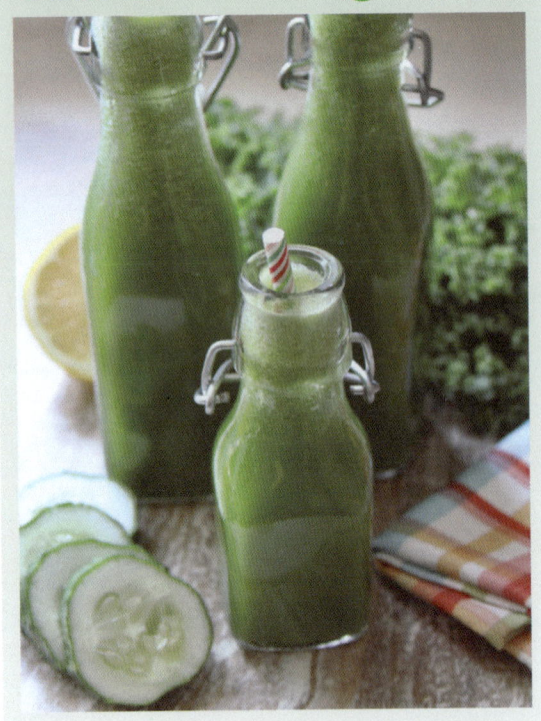

### Ingredients

- 12 small leaves Thai basil
- 1 handful Italian parsley
- 1/2 inch ginger
- 1 large orange, peeled
- 1/2 lemon
- 3 cups spinach
- 1/2 cucumber
- 2 apples
- 2 pieces celery
- 1 cup grapes

*Yield: 30 ounces*

# DAY 12

## Orange Theory

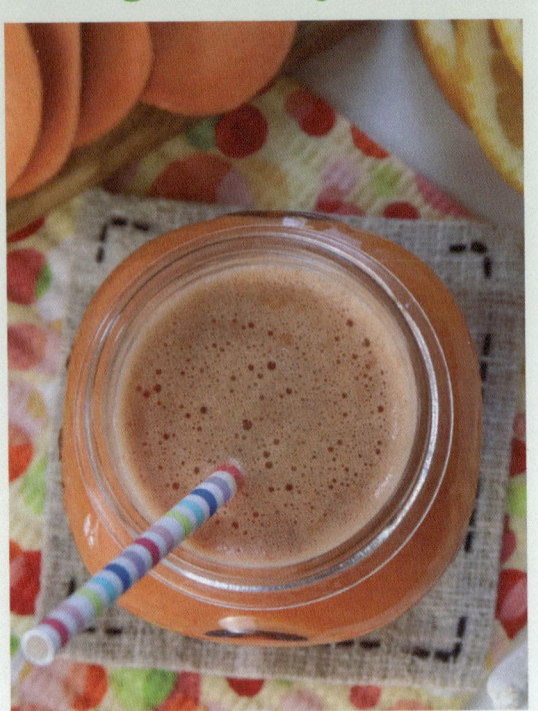

### Ingredients

- 2 sweet potatoes
- 2 apples
- 2 oranges, peeled
- 2 celery
- 1 inch ginger
- 1 dash cinnamon

*Yield: 32 ounces*

# DAY 13

## Green Cheer

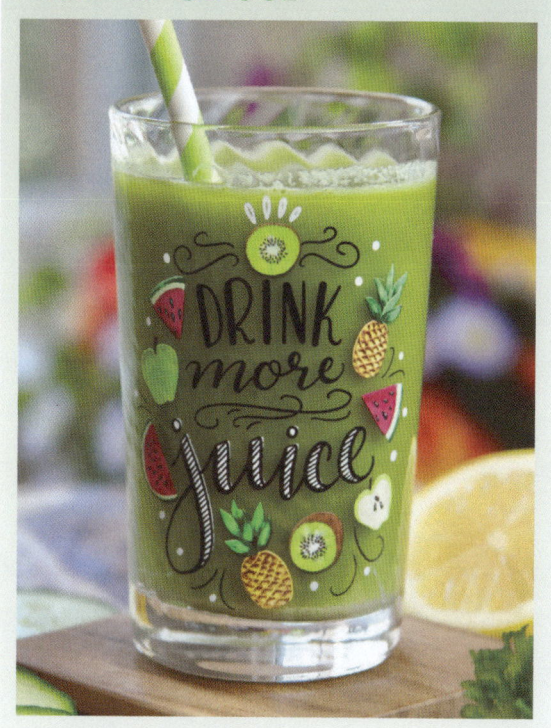

### Ingredients

- 2 apples
- 1 cucumber
- 1 inch ginger
- 1/2 lemon
- 1 orange, peeled
- 1 handful parsley
- 2 cups spinach
- 1 avocado (blended into the juice)

Yield: 30 ounces

# DAY 14

## Heart Beet

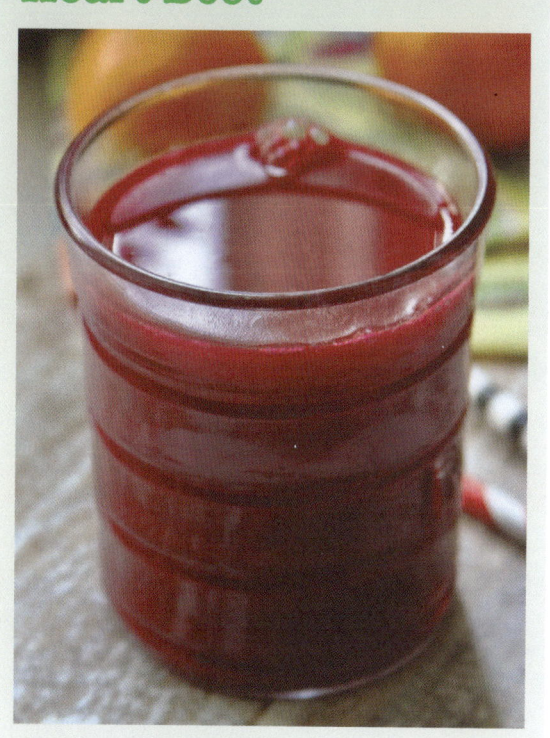

### Ingredients

- 1 apple
- 1 beet
- 12 carrots
- 1/2 lemon
- 2 oranges, peeled

Yield: 32 ounces

**Yield**
30 ounces

*A fellow juicer wrote in and said he was about to give up on juicing when he tried this recipe. He enjoyed it so much he decided to renew his commitment to juicing. I thought it was the perfect recipe for renewal week!*

# Day 8: The Anytime Cocktail

## Ingredients

- 2 apples
- 2 celery
- 1 cucumber
- 5 kale leaves
- 1/2 lemon
- 2 oranges, peeled
- 1 handful parsley

*"Find something you're passionate about, and keep tremendously interested in it."*

— Julia Child

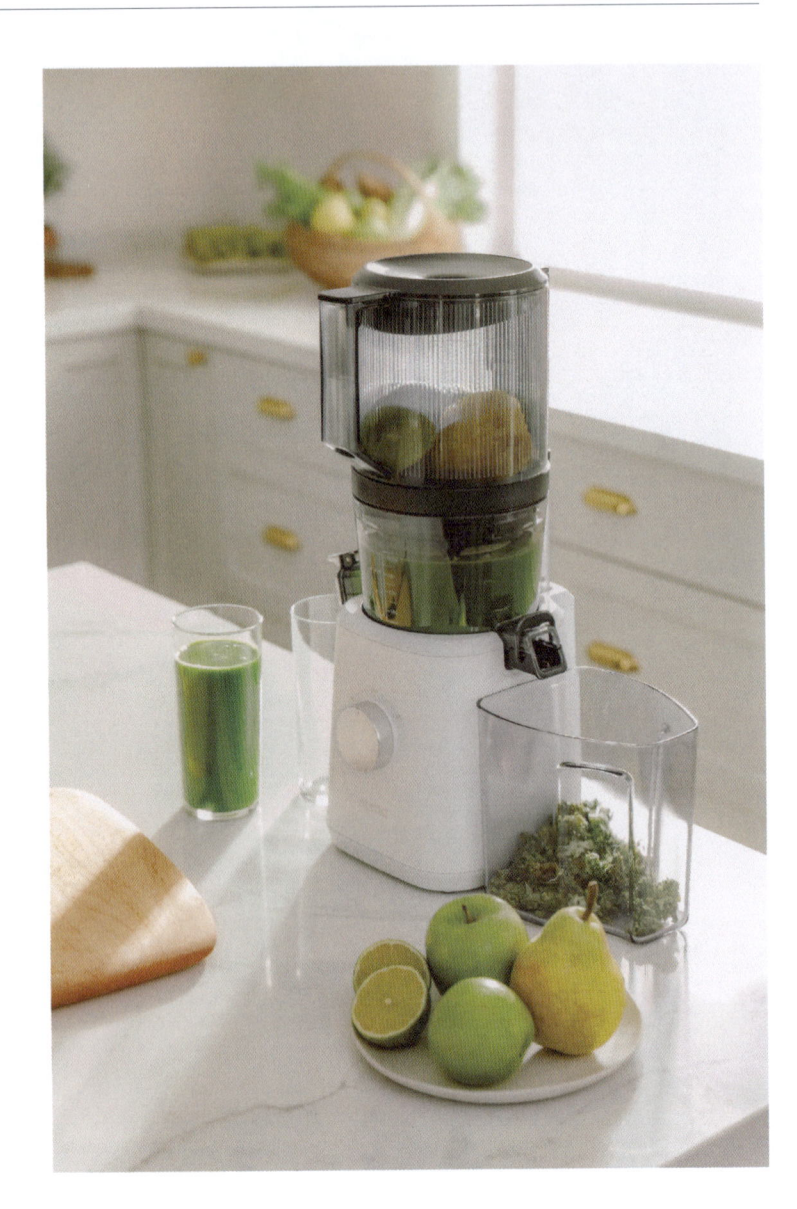

**Yield**
32 ounces

*This juice is Joe Cross's from his movie* **Fat, Sick and Nearly Dead**. *If you haven't seen this film, I highly recommend it and found his journey to be inspiring and life changing!*

# Day 9: Mean Green

## Ingredients

- 2 apples
- 4 celery
- 1 cucumber
- 1 inch ginger
- 6 kale leaves
- 1/2 lemon

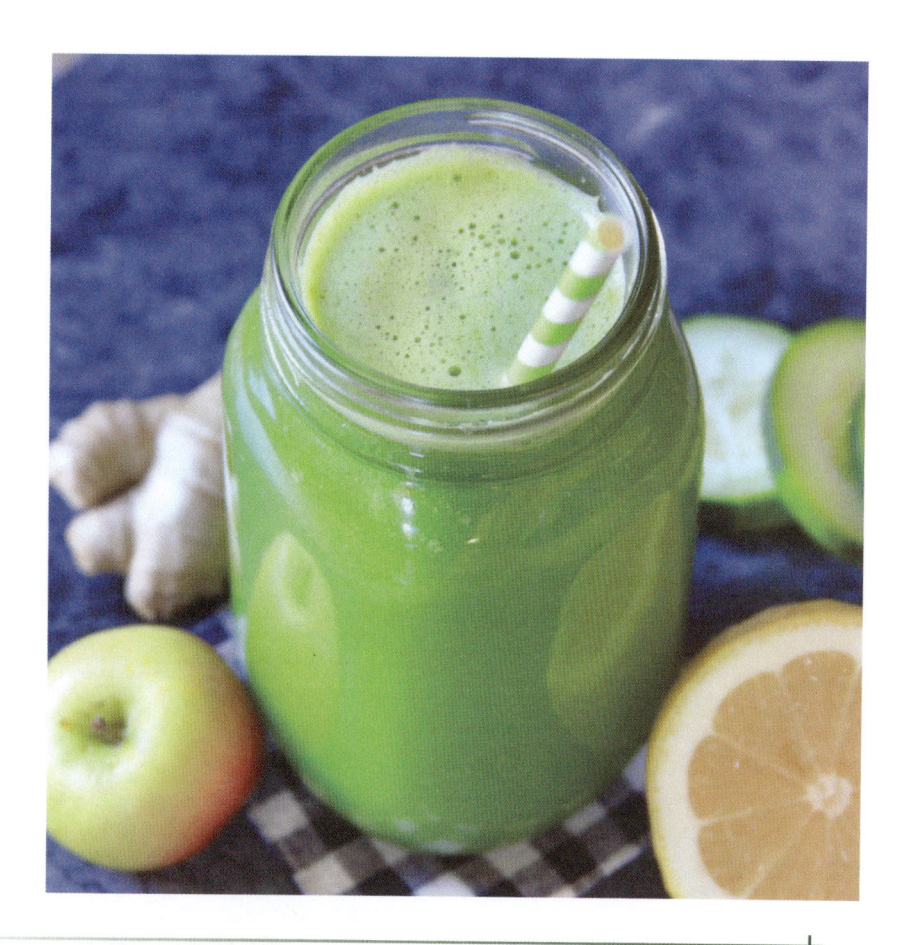

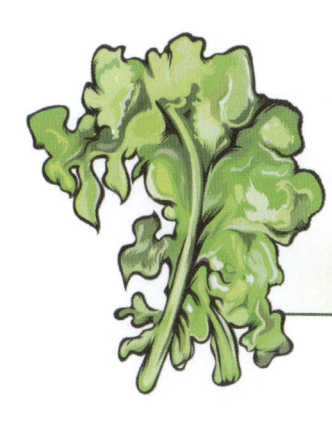

*If you have a high speed centrifugal juicer and are having trouble getting the greens to process, you can sandwich the kale between pieces of apple to get a slightly better yield from the kale.*

**Yield**
30 ounces

*This recipe is a perfect beginner juice. Parents have written that they have used this recipe for their kids who wouldn't touch a fruit or a vegetable.*

# Day 10: Apple Crisp

## Ingredients

- 5 apples
- 2 oranges, peeled
- 2 celery

"Either you run the day, or the day runs you."

— Jim Rohn

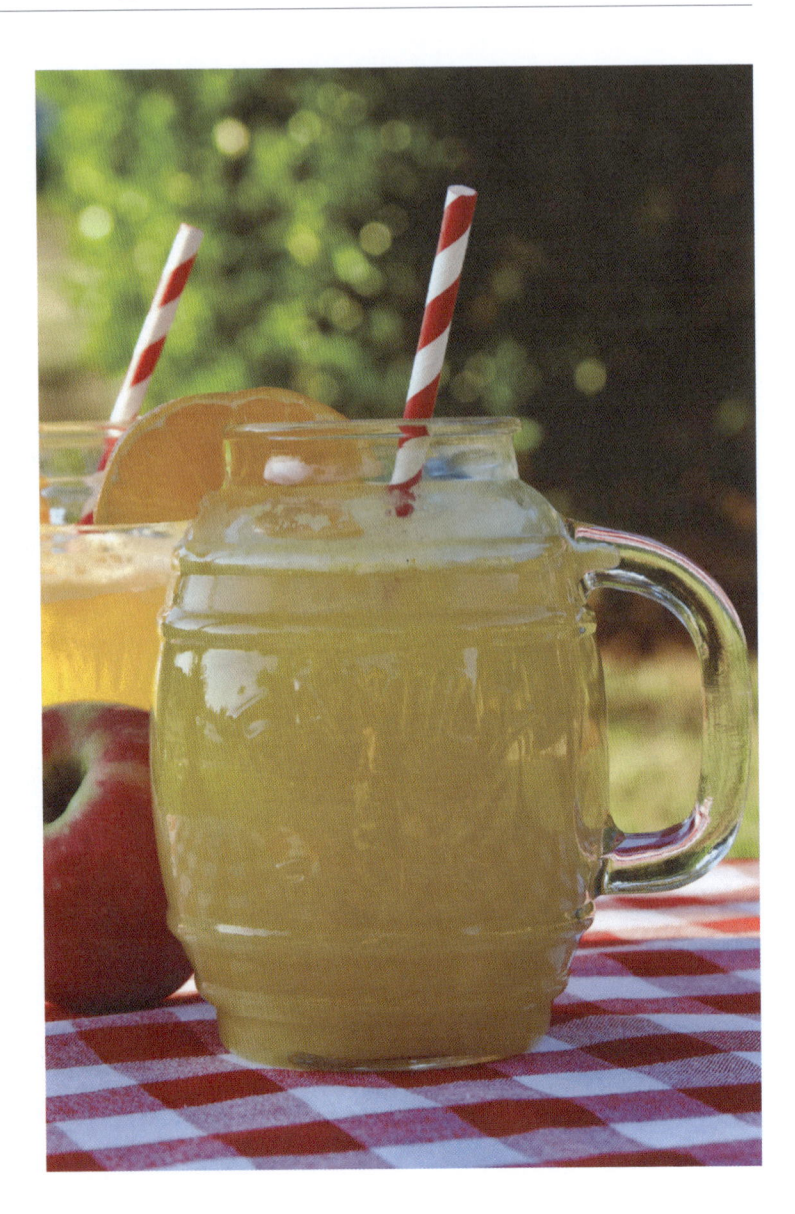

**Yield**
30 ounces

*If you do not have Thai basil, regular basil works well in this recipe also.*

# Day 11: Thai Green Magic

## Ingredients

- 12 small leaves Thai basil
- 1 handful Italian parsley
- 1/2 inch ginger
- 1 orange, peeled
- 1/2 lemon
- 3 cups spinach
- 1/2 cucumber
- 2 apples
- 2 pieces celery
- 1 cup grapes

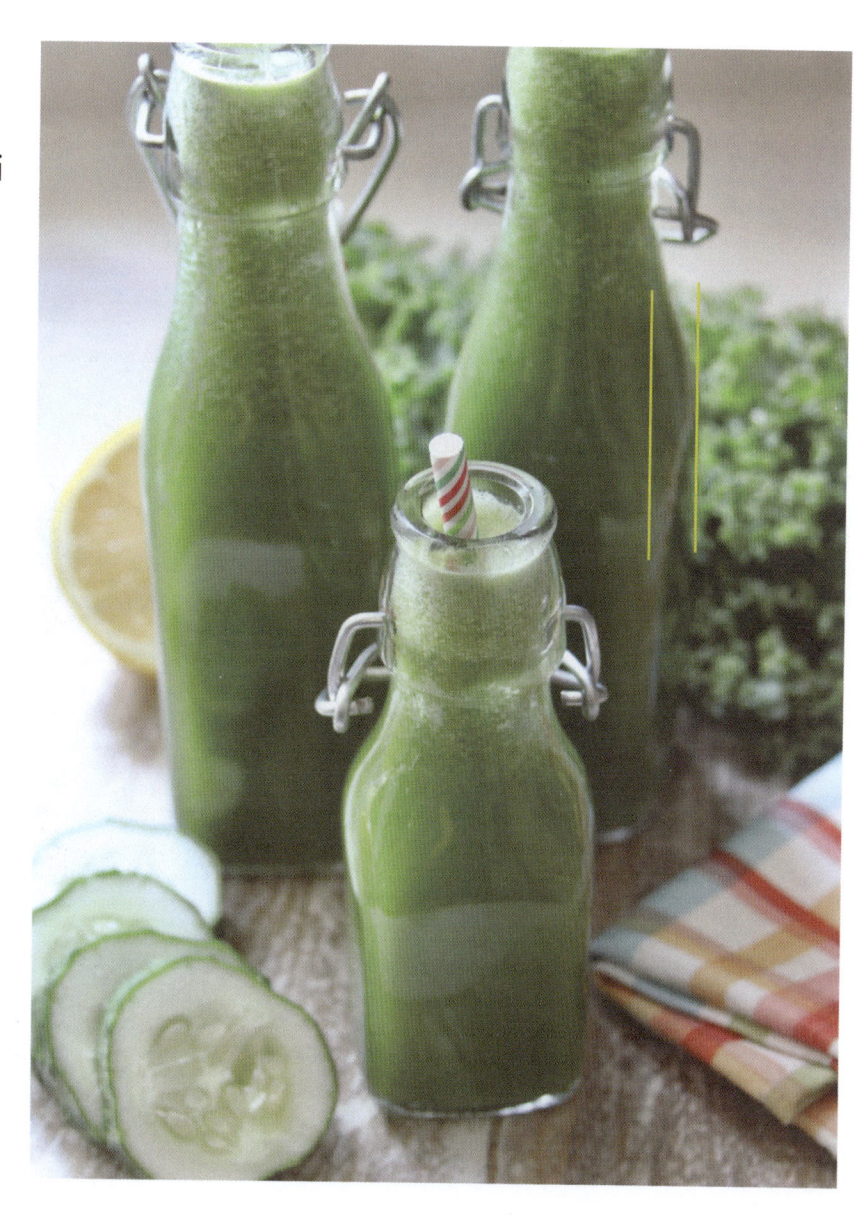

**Yield**
32 ounces

*Sweet potatoes add a nice, satiny texture to the juice. They help stabilize blood sugar, enhance brain function, are high in antioxidants and are good for eye health.*

# Day 12: Orange Theory

## Ingredients

- 2 sweet potatoes
- 2 apples
- 2 oranges, peeled
- 2 celery
- 1 inch ginger
- 1 dash cinnamon

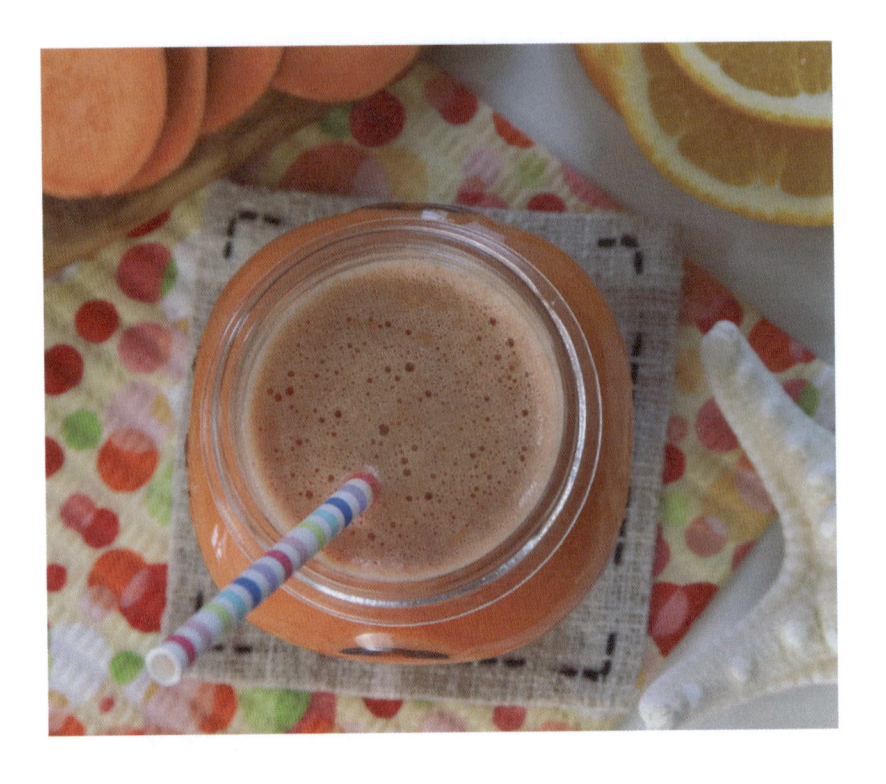

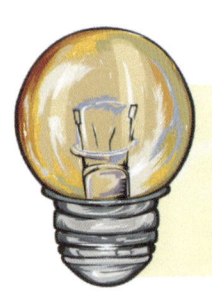

*Sweet potato should be juiced raw and does not need to be peeled unless it contains unappetizing spots.*

**Yield**
30 ounces

This juice works very well as a meal replacement. The avocado gives the juice a smooth texture and makes it more filling.

# Day 13: Green Cheer

## Ingredients

- 2 apples
- 1 cucumber
- 1 inch ginger
- 1/2 lemon
- 1 orange, peeled
- 1 handful parsley
- 2 cups spinach
- 1 avocado (blended into the juice)

**Directions:** Juice all ingredients together except for the avocado. Blend avocado into the juice with a blender.

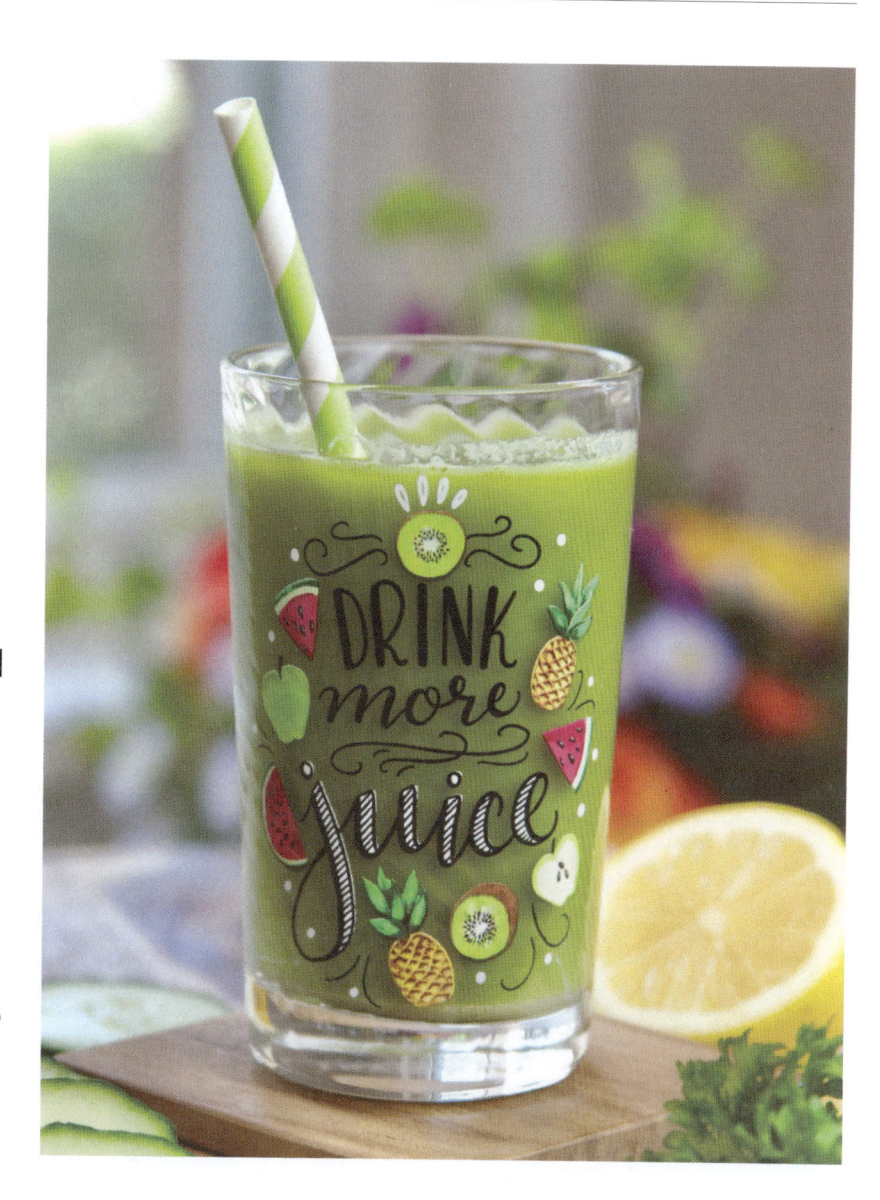

The Challenge: Days 8-14

**Yield**
32 ounces

*This juice also tastes delicious with an inch of fresh ginger. You do not need to peel the ginger for juicing, as the peel goes into the pulp bin.*

# Day 14: Heart Beet

## Ingredients

- 1 apple
- 1 beet
- 12 carrots
- 1/2 lemon
- 2 oranges, peeled

"My goal is not to be better than anyone else, but to be better than I used to be."

— Wayne Dyer

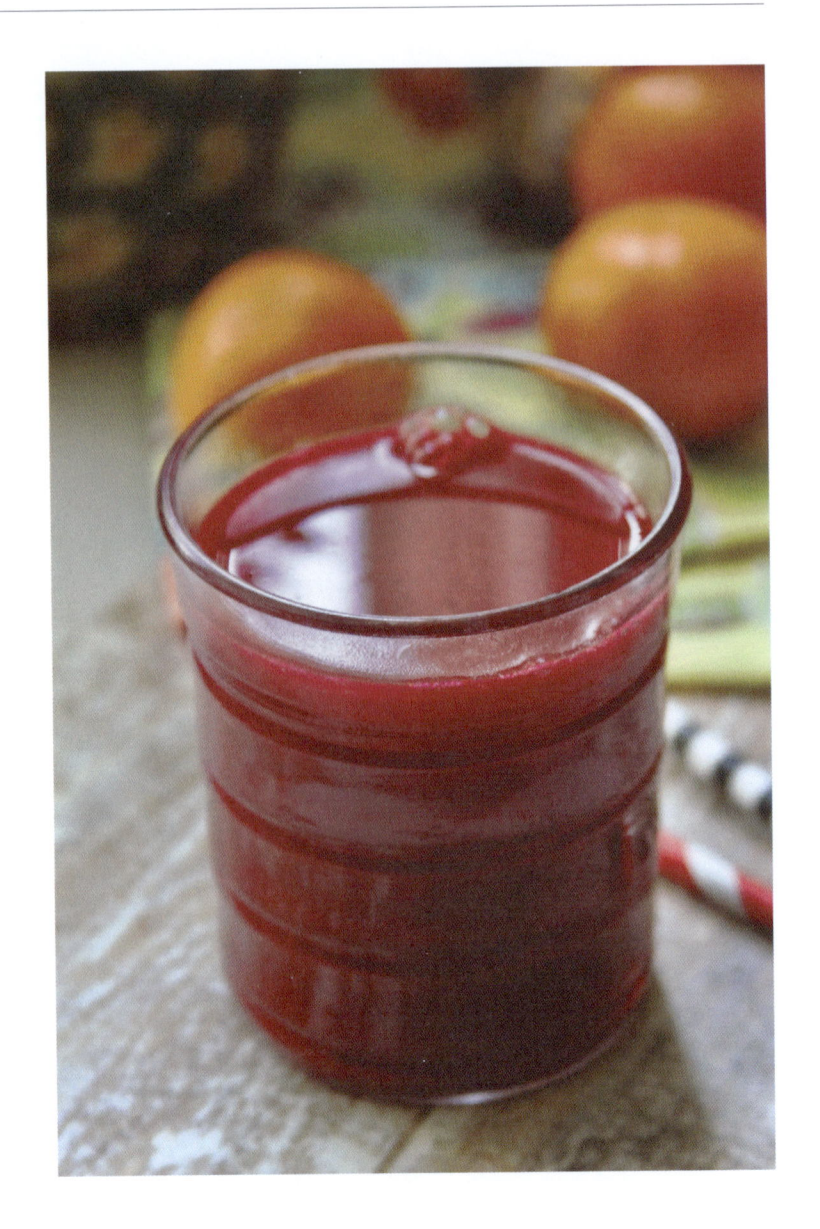

# Days 8-14 Assessment

What were my strongest points this week?
_____
_____
_____


Did I juice or have juice every day of the challenge?_____

What was my favorite recipe? _____

Were there any unexpected obstacles? If so, how did I handle them with regards to juicing?
_____
_____
_____


Is there anything I can do to prepare for next week to make it even better?
_____
_____
_____

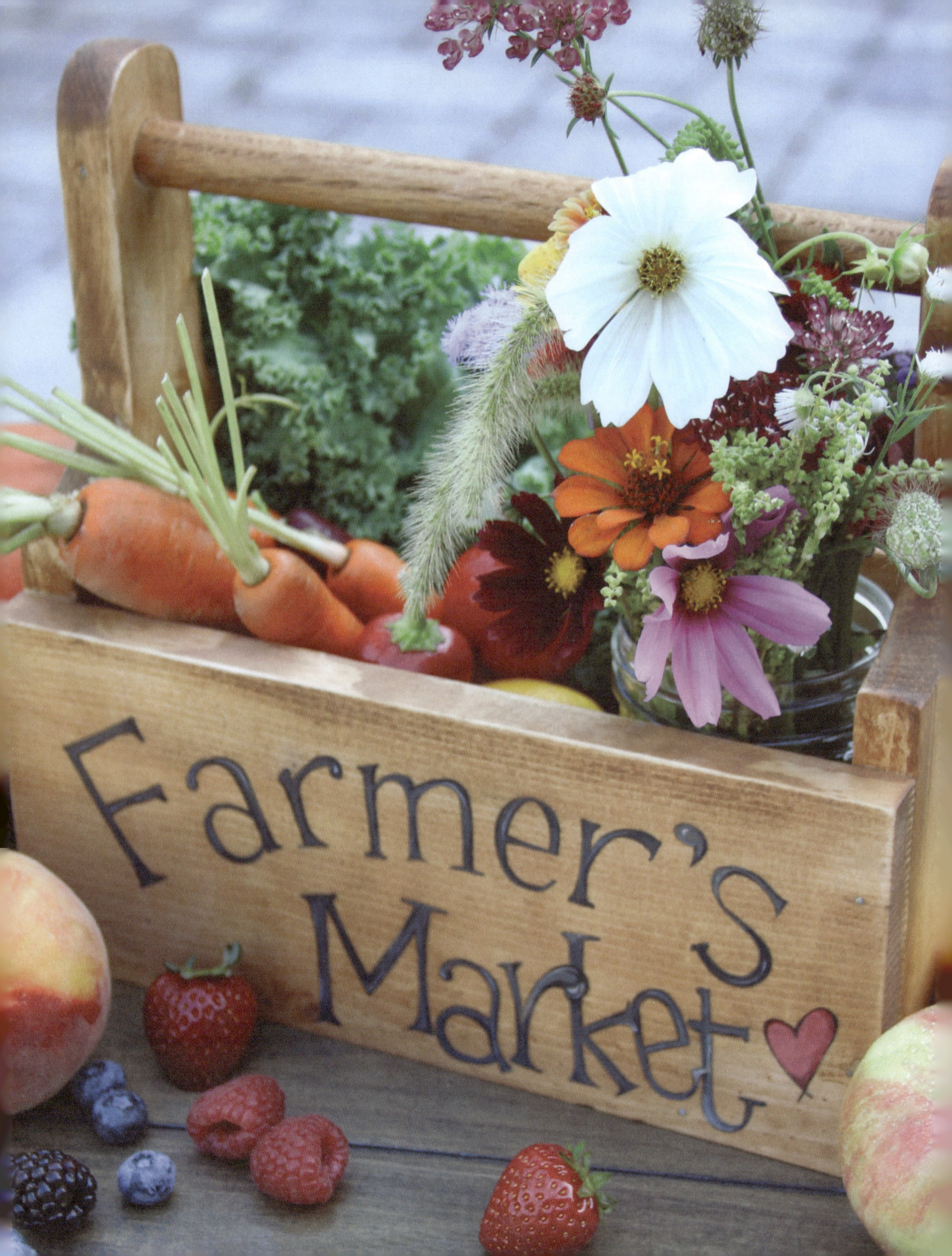

# Days 15-21 Shopping List

**Beet Week!** The third week contains a few recipes that contain beets. If the greens are still attached to the beetroot, you can juice them — as they are an excellent source of iron, vitamins and other minerals.

## Vegetables
- [ ] 3 beets
- [ ] 33 carrots
- [ ] 10 pieces celery
- [ ] 2 cucumbers
- [ ] 1 sweet potato
- [ ] 1 zucchini

## Fruits
- [ ] 14 apples
- [ ] 5 lemons
- [ ] 1 lime
- [ ] 5 oranges
- [ ] 4 pears
- [ ] 1 1/2 cups strawberries

## Herbs & Spices
- [ ] black pepper
- [ ] cinnamon
- [ ] 5 inches ginger
- [ ] 1 teaspoon honey
- [ ] 19 mint leaves
- [ ] 6 inches turmeric
- [ ] 1 cup white or green tea

Just a reminder that the 30 day challenge is not a cleanse, but rather 30 days of recipes designed to help incorporate juicing into daily life.

As you approach this new week, do you feel better than you did seven days ago? Are you becoming more efficient at juicing and cleaning the juicer?

Sometimes I play my favorite songs to create an atmosphere in the kitchen and make juicing more enjoyable.

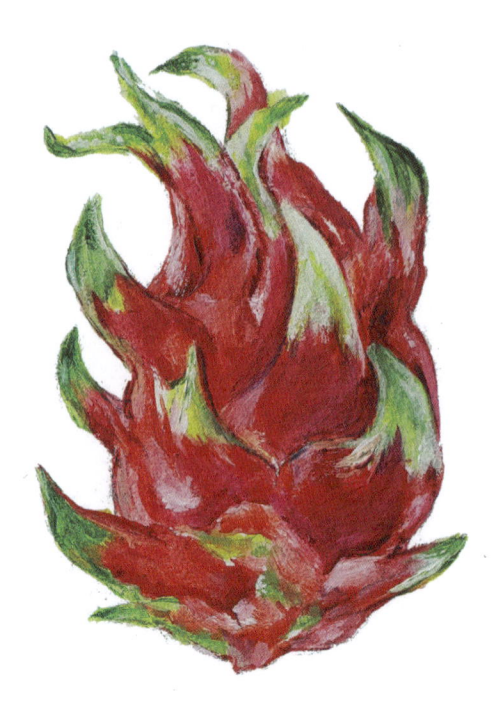

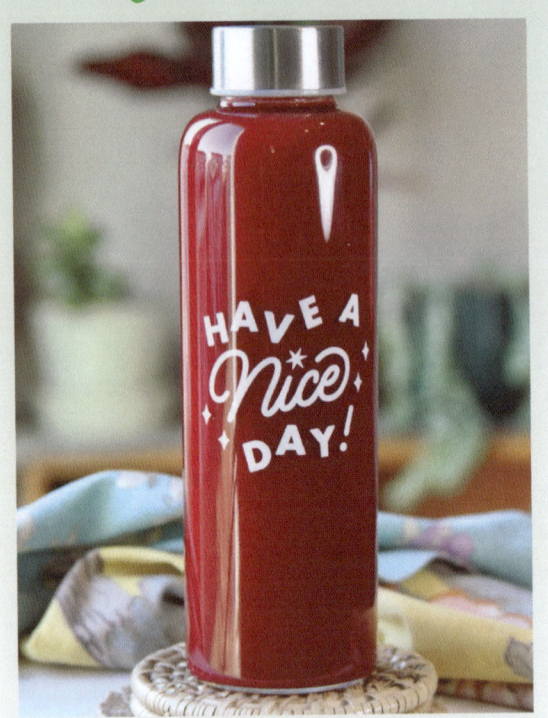

# DAY 15
## Candy Crush

### Ingredients
- 2 apples
- 1 beet
- 6 carrots
- 2 celery
- 1/2 cucumber
- 1 inch ginger
- 1/2 lemon
- 1 orange, peeled

*Yield: 32 ounces*

# DAY 16

## Green Ginger Ale

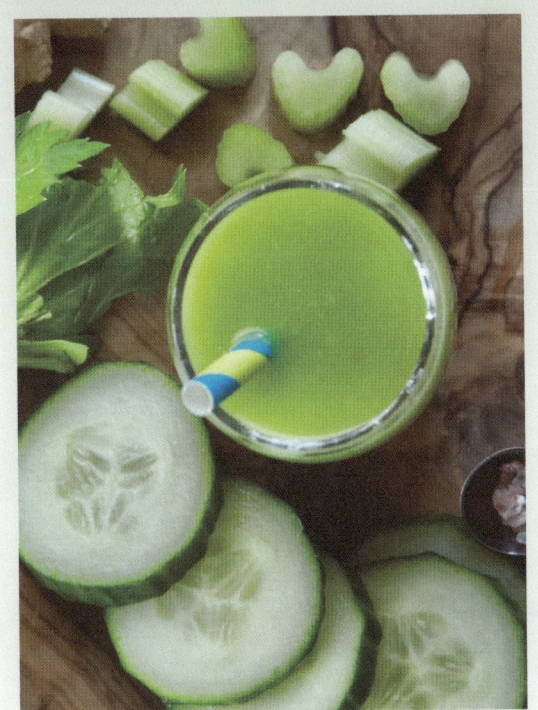

### Ingredients

- 3 apples
- 2 celery
- 1 cucumber
- 1 inch ginger
- 1 lime

Yield: 28 ounces

# DAY 17

## The Accelerator

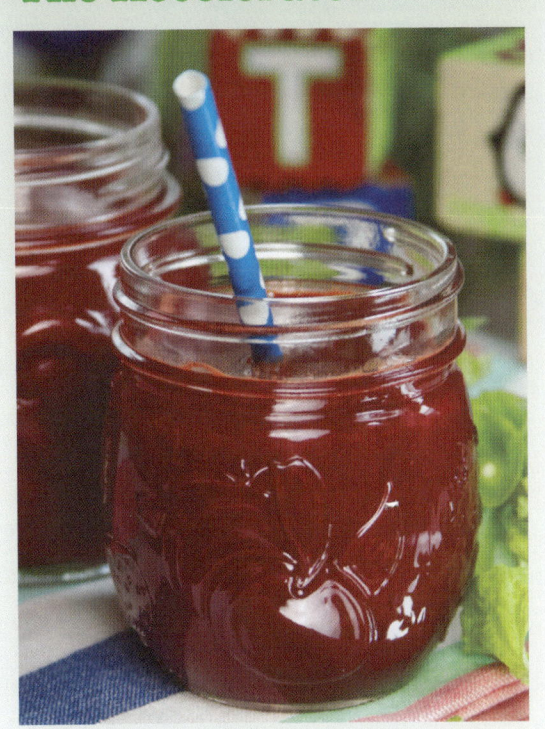

### Ingredients

- 1 apple
- 1 beet
- 1 dash black pepper
- 5 carrots
- 1 celery
- 1 dash cinnamon
- 1 inch ginger
- 1/2 lemon
- 1 orange, peeled
- 1 sweet potato
- 1 zucchini

Yield: 32 ounces

# DAY 18

## Turmeric Sunrise

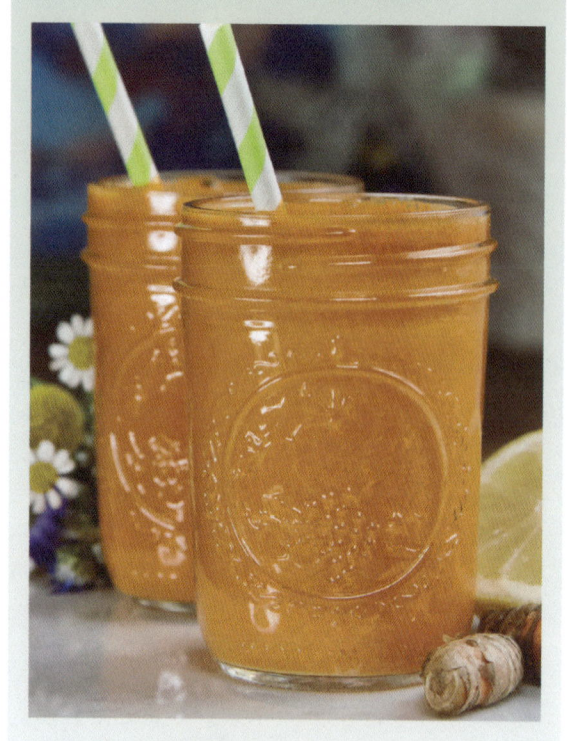

### Ingredients

- 2 apples
- 3 carrots
- 3 celery
- 1 inch ginger
- 2 lemons, peeled
- 2 pears
- 6 inches turmeric (or 1 teaspoon powdered)

Yield: 30 ounces

# DAY 19

## Cinnamint

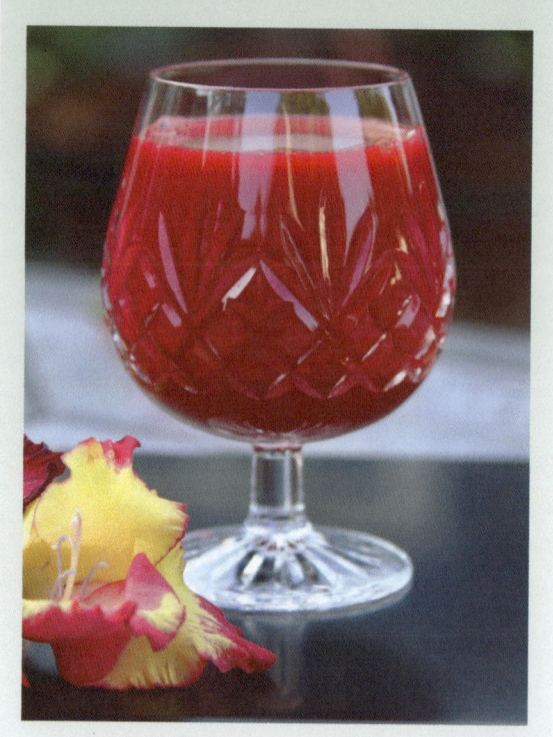

### Ingredients

- 7 mint leaves
- 1 beet
- 1 lemon
- 5 carrots
- 2 pieces celery
- 1 orange, peeled
- 2 apples
- 2 pears
- 1/2 inch ginger
- 1/4 teaspoon cinnamon

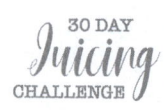

Yield: 32 ounces

# DAY 20

## Strawberry Mint Julep

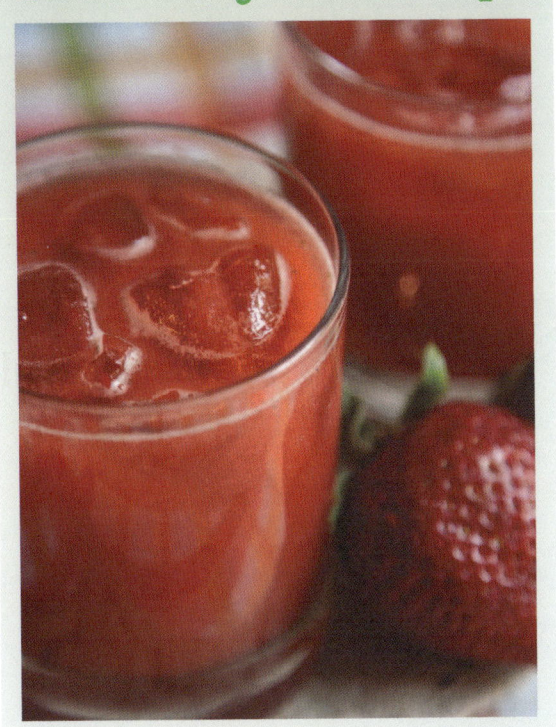

### Ingredients

- 2 apples
- 1 cup white or green tea, chilled
- 1 1/2 cups strawberries
- 1/4 lemon
- 1 teaspoon honey
- 12 mint leaves

*Yield: 28 ounces*

# DAY 21

## The Eye Opener

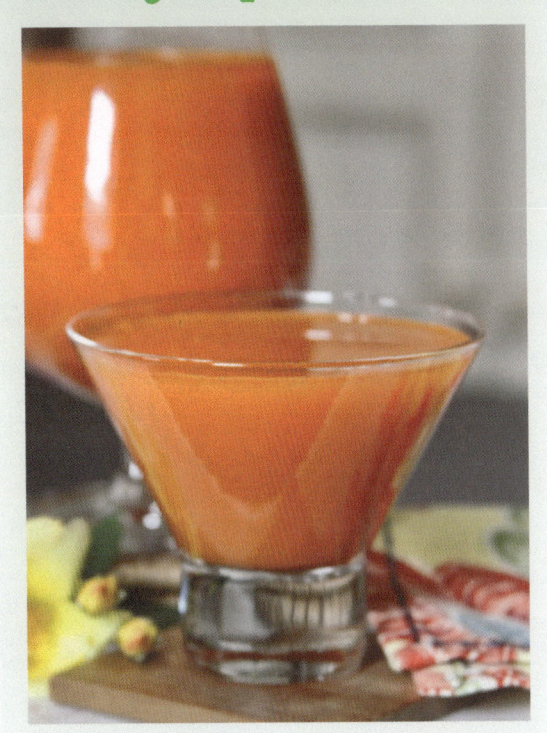

### Ingredients

- 2 apples
- 14 carrots
- 2 oranges, peeled

*Yield: 32 ounces*

**Yield**
32 ounces

*As you begin the second half of your challenge, may you find yourself feeling stronger and more energetic with each passing day. The first recipe of this week is one of my favorites! I hope you enjoy it too.*

## Day 15: Candy Crush

### Ingredients

- 2 apples
- 1 beet
- 6 carrots
- 2 celery
- 1/2 cucumber
- 1 inch ginger
- 1/2 lemon
- 1 orange, peeled

"The first step towards getting somewhere is to decide that you are not going to stay where you are."

— J. Pierpont

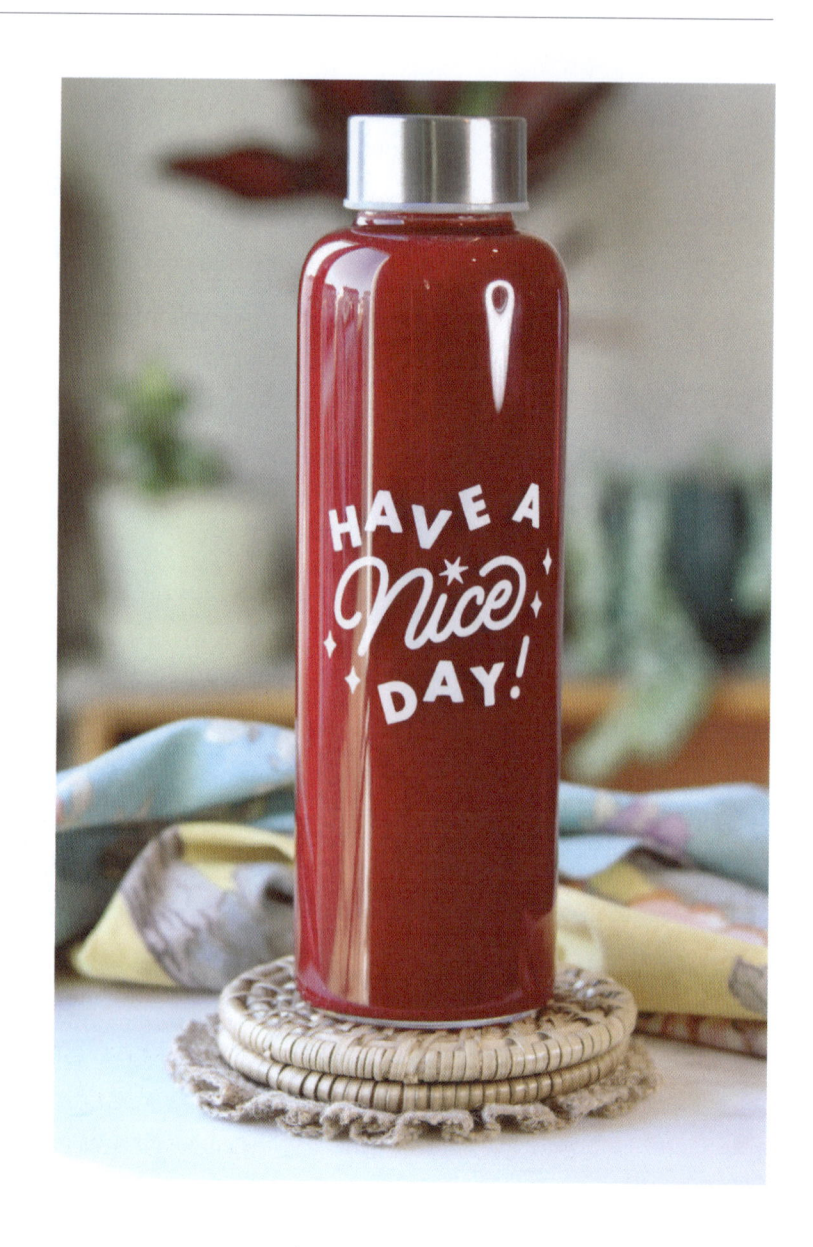

**Yield**
28 ounces

This recipe is wonderful for the skin. Cucumbers are good for maintaining healthy hair, skin and nails.

# Day 16: Green Ginger Ale

## Ingredients

- 3 apples
- 2 celery
- 1 cucumber
- 1 inch ginger
- 1 lime

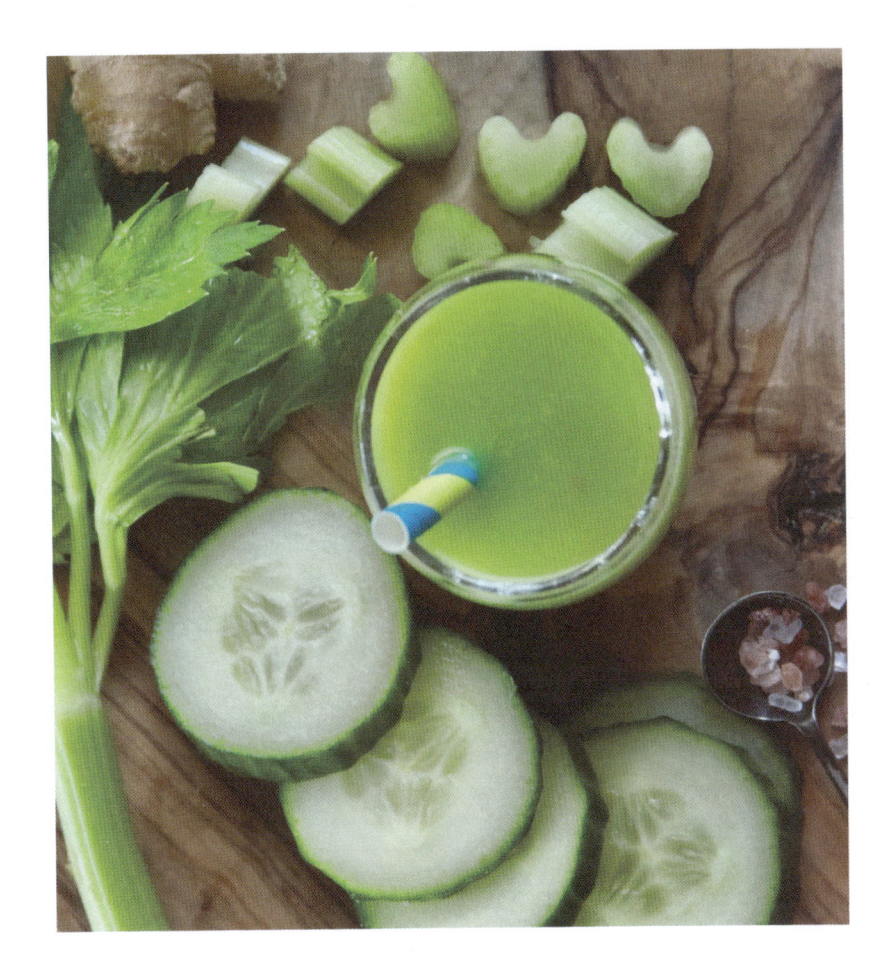

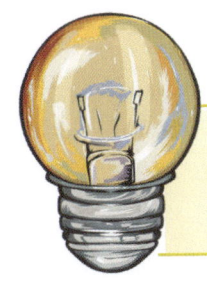

You do not need to peel the lime when juicing, but the peeling will make the juice slightly more tart.

The Challenge: Days 15-21

**Yield**
32 ounces

This recipe is an excellent weight loss juice. Cinnamon is a good fat burner, and beets are helpful in cleansing the liver. One of the liver's many functions is processing fat, and cleansing the liver is important for natural weight loss.

# Day 17: The Accelerator

## Ingredients
- 1 apple
- 1 beet
- 1 dash black pepper
- 5 carrots
- 1 celery
- 1 dash cinnamon
- 1 inch ginger
- 1/2 lemon
- 1 orange, peeled
- 1 sweet potato
- 1 zucchini

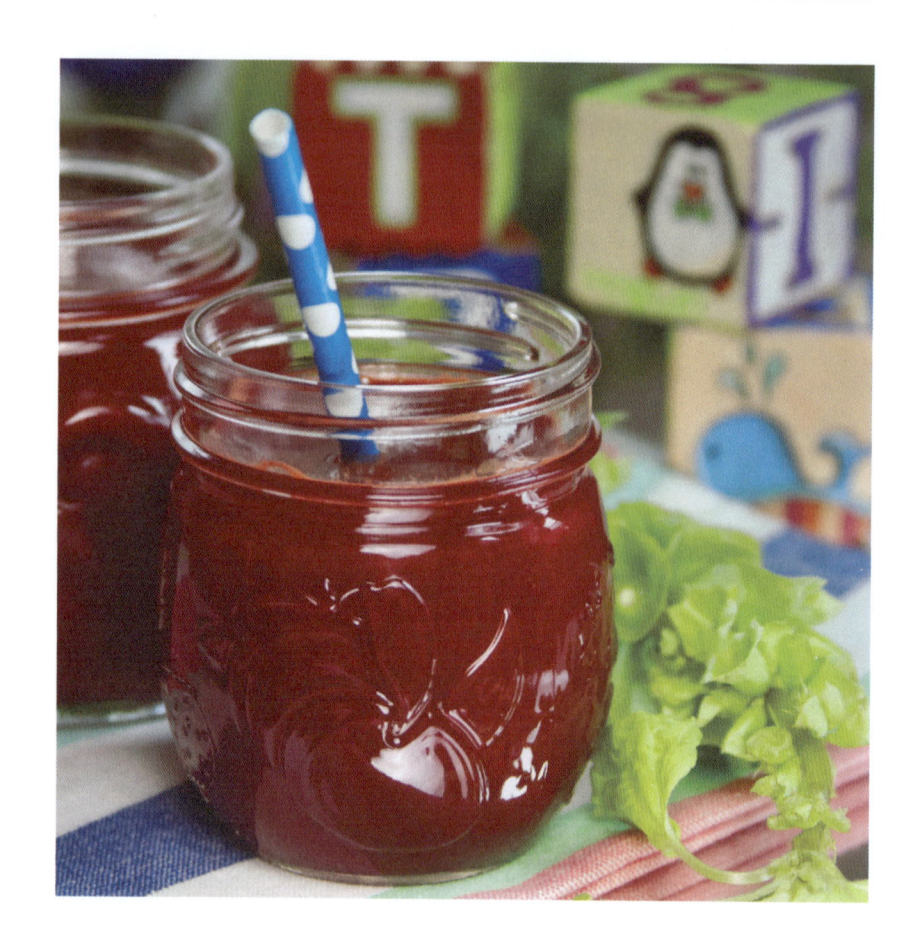

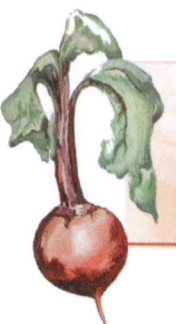

Do juice the greens that are attached to the beet, as they are loaded with vitamins and minerals and often contain more iron than the beetroot itself.

**Yield**
30 ounces

As mentioned earlier, adding freshly cracked pepper helps the body's ability to utilize the turmeric. This recipe is also delicious with fresh mint leaves.

# Day 18: Turmeric Sunrise

## Ingredients

- 2 apples
- 3 carrots
- 3 celery
- 1 inch ginger
- 2 lemons, peeled
- 2 pears
- 6 inches turmeric (or 1 teaspoon powdered)

"Every day is a renewal, every morning the daily miracle. This joy you feel is life."

— Gertrude Stein

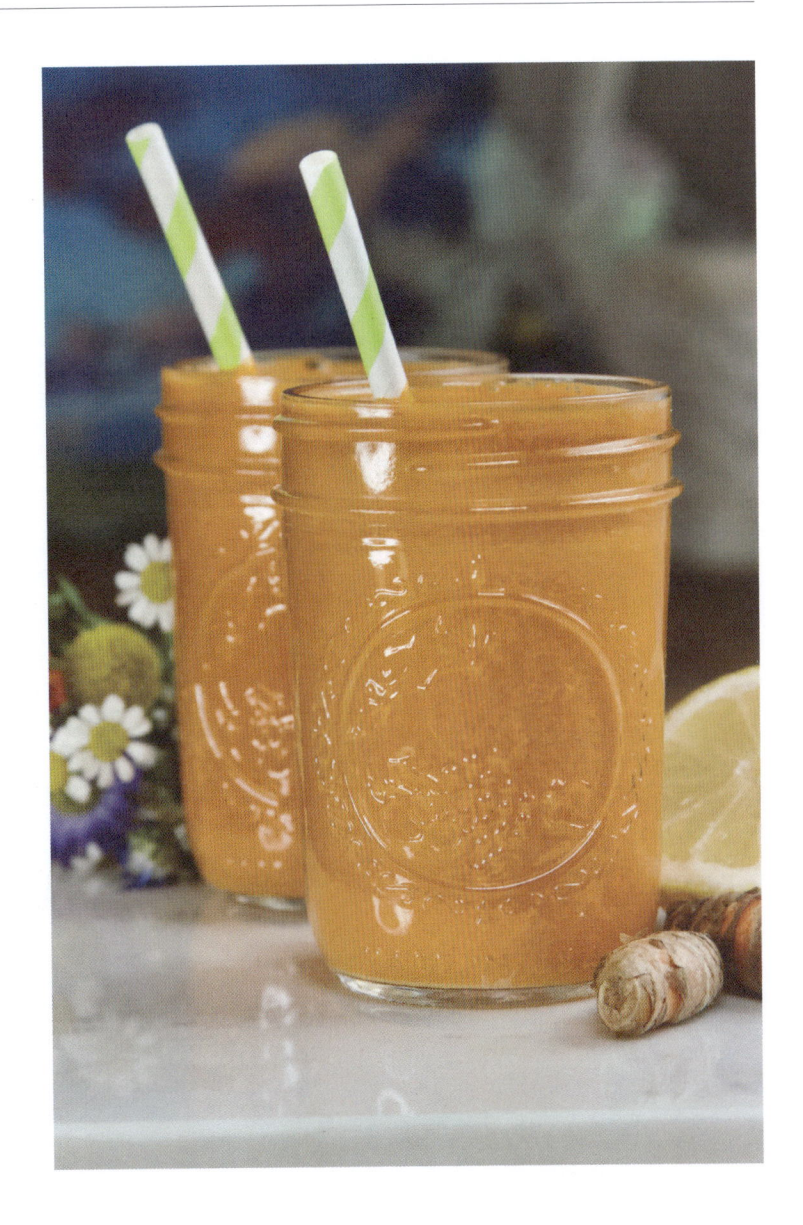

The Challenge: Days 15-21    61

**Yield**
32 ounces

*The combination of ingredients in this recipe gives it a unique flavor all its own.*

# Day 19: Cinnamint

## Ingredients

- 7 mint leaves
- 1 beet
- 1 lemon
- 5 carrots
- 2 pieces celery
- 1 orange, peeled
- 2 apples
- 2 pears
- 1/2 inch ginger
- 1/4 teaspoon cinnamon

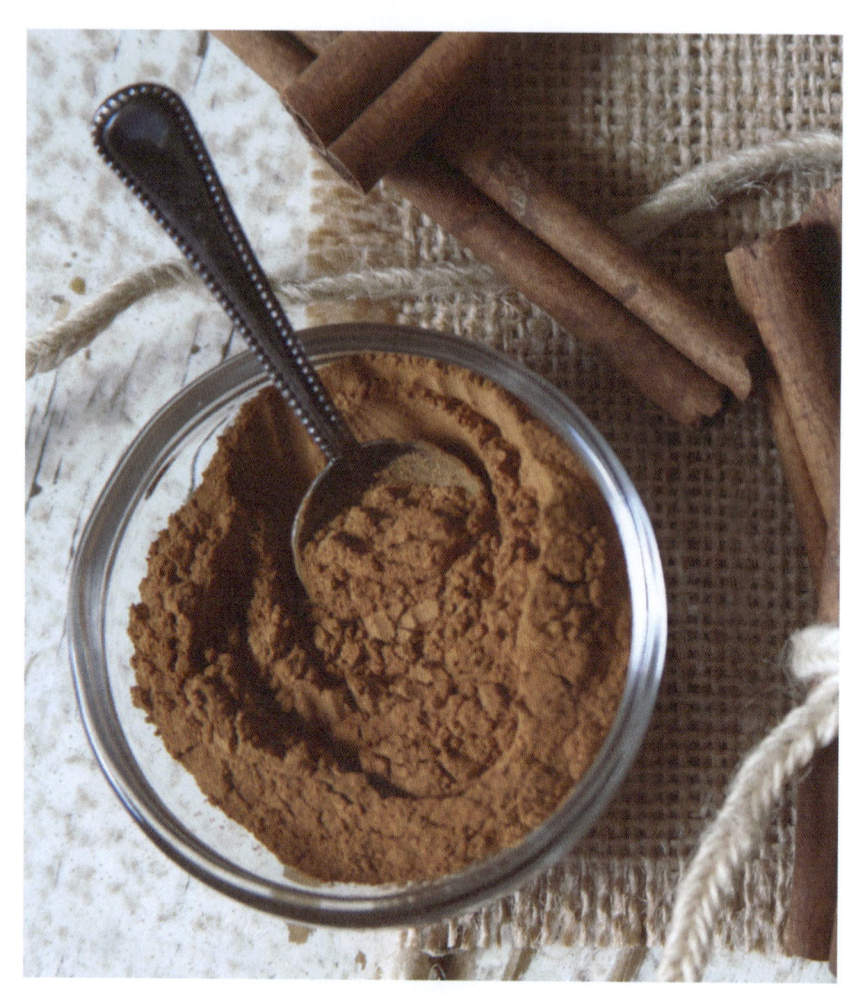

*Cinnamon provides antioxidants, vitamins, minerals and has been used around the world for thousands of years as a healing aid.*

**Yield**
28 ounces

*This recipe is perfect for company and to share with others who have never juiced before. One of my friends tried it and said it tasted too good to be healthy!*

# Day 20: Strawberry Mint Julep

## Ingredients

- 2 apples
- 1 cup white or green tea, chilled
- 1 1/2 cups strawberries
- 1/4 lemon
- 1 teaspoon honey
- 12 mint leaves

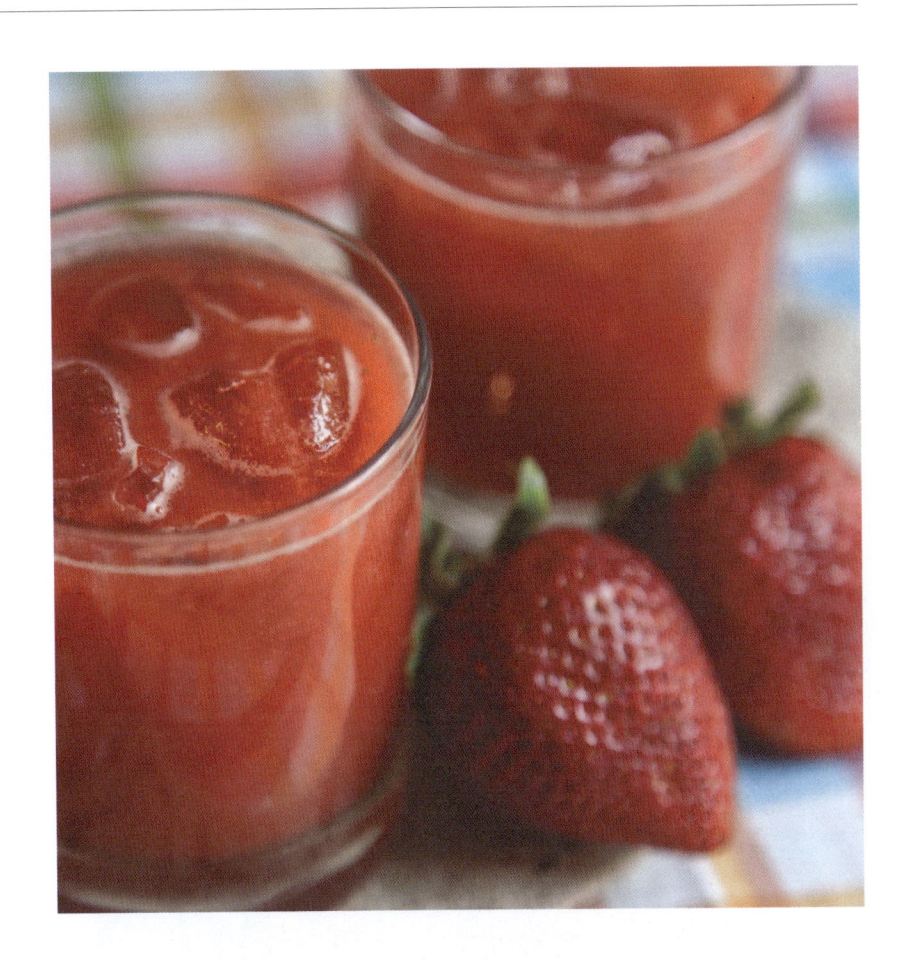

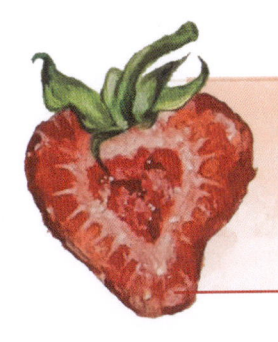

**Directions:** Steep a cup of white tea, add honey and let it cool. Juice the produce and mint leaves. Pour cooled tea into juice and serve over ice.

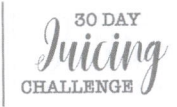

**Yield**
32 ounces

*We're already at the end of week three! I find it motivating to imagine all the vitamins, minerals and enzymes entering into my bloodstream and traveling where they are needed most in my body. What inspires you to juice?*

# Day 21: The Eye Opener

## Ingredients

- 2 apples
- 14 carrots
- 2 oranges, peeled

"Determine what you want and why you want it. Once you understand what's important, you can utilize your passions and achieve anything."

— Brooke Griffin

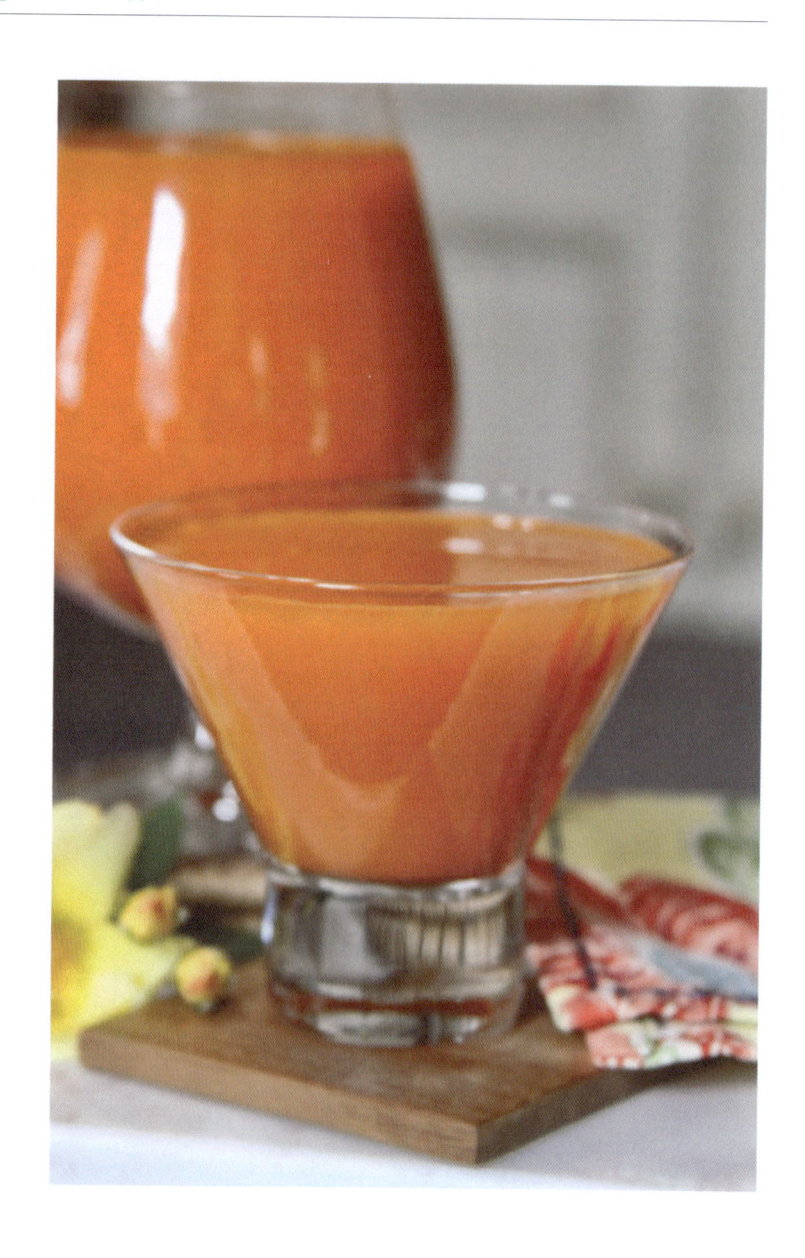

# Days 15-21 Assessment

What were my strongest points this week?

_____
_____
_____

Did I juice or have juice every day of the challenge? _____

What was my favorite recipe? _____

Were there any unexpected obstacles? If so, how did I handle them with regards to juicing?

_____
_____
_____

Is there anything I can do to prepare for next week to make it even better?

_____
_____
_____

Farmer's Market
*leeks*

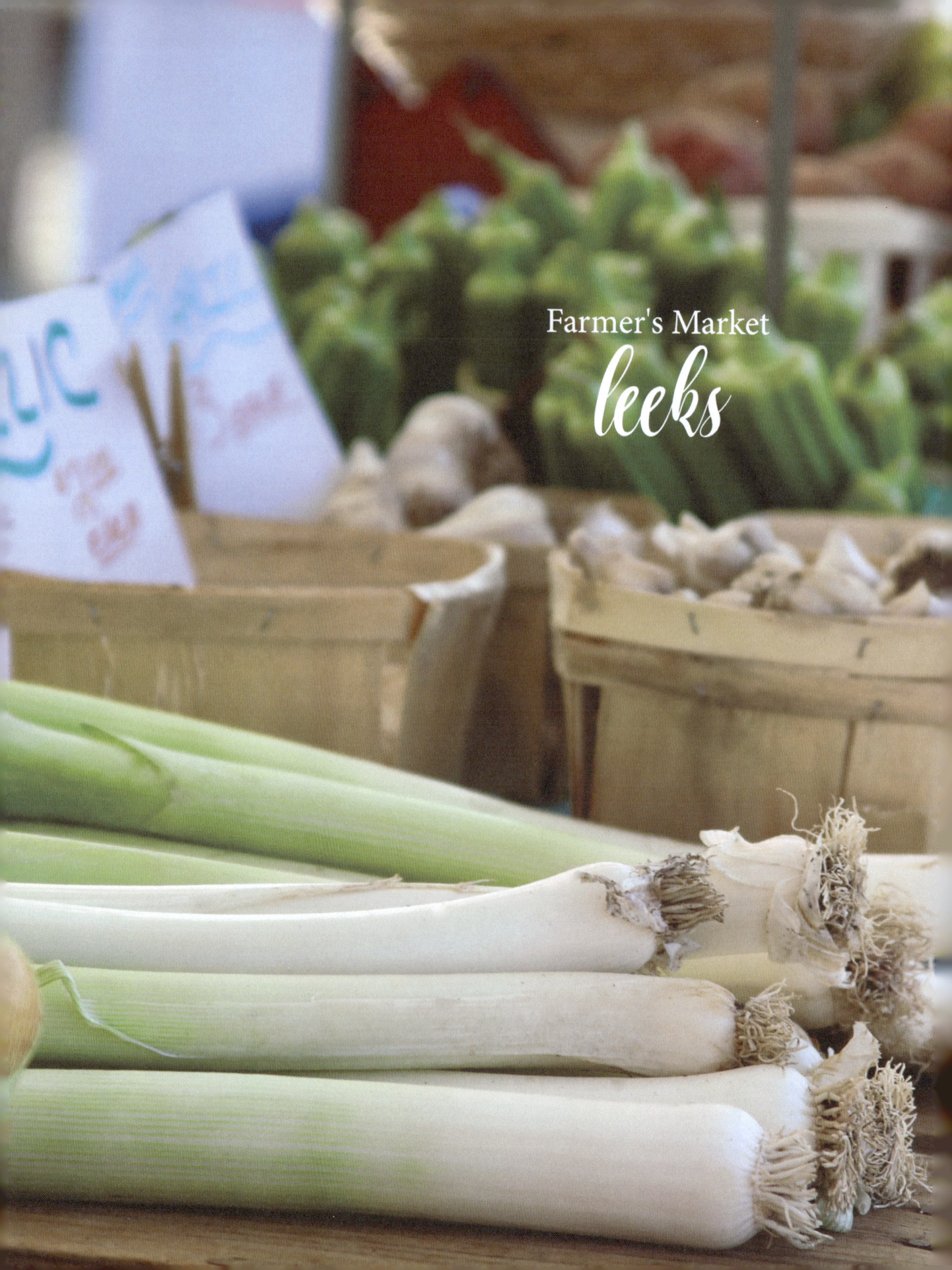

# Days 22-28 Shopping List

**Pineapple Week!** This seven days has a few delicious recipes containing pineapple. Not only are pineapples an international symbol for hospitality, they also have properties that may help reduce inflammation and pain.

## Vegetables

- [ ] 1 avocado
- [ ] 1 beet
- [ ] 14 carrots
- [ ] 4 pieces celery
- [ ] 2 cucumbers
- [ ] 3 kale leaves
- [ ] 3 cups spinach
- [ ] 2 sweet potatoes
- [ ] 1 zucchini

## Fruits

- [ ] 8 apples
- [ ] 3 lemons
- [ ] 1 lime
- [ ] 3 oranges
- [ ] 3 pears
- [ ] 9 1/2 cups pineapple

## Herbs & Spices

- [ ] cayenne pepper
- [ ] 1 fennel bulb
- [ ] 9 inches ginger
- [ ] 10 mint leaves
- [ ] 1 bunch parsley

Some experts believe it takes only 21 days to create a habit. Whether this is true for you or not, you are definitely well on your way!

Have you established a routine? Do you find yourself looking forward to the next juice? Sometimes when I make two of my recipes ahead of time, I have to juice again for the following day because I'll drink both days' recipes on the day I made it. Has this been the case for you also?

Hope you are feeling stronger and more energetic each day!

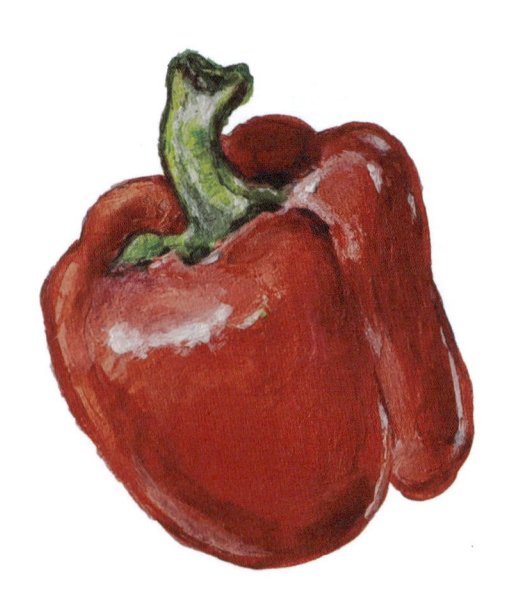

# DAY 22
## Sweet Adeline

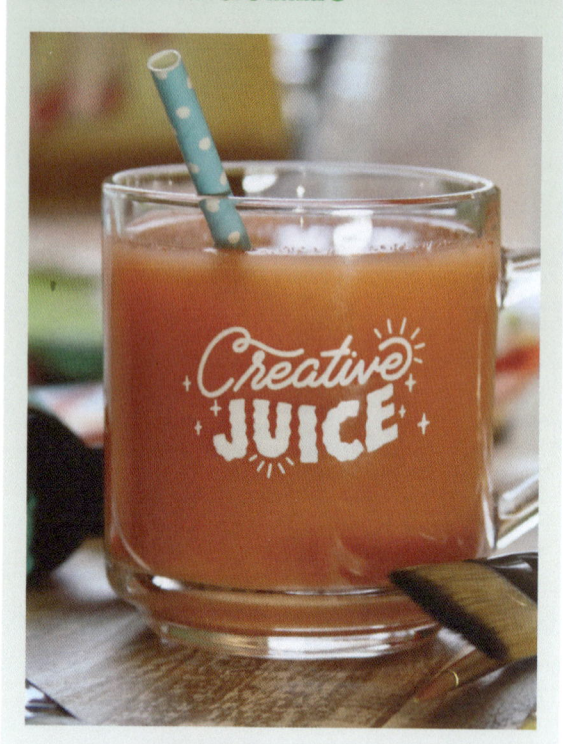

### Ingredients
- 2 apples
- 6 carrots
- 2 pieces celery
- 1 inch ginger
- 2 cups pineapple
- 1 sweet potato

*Yield: 30 ounces*

# DAY 23
## Fennelicious

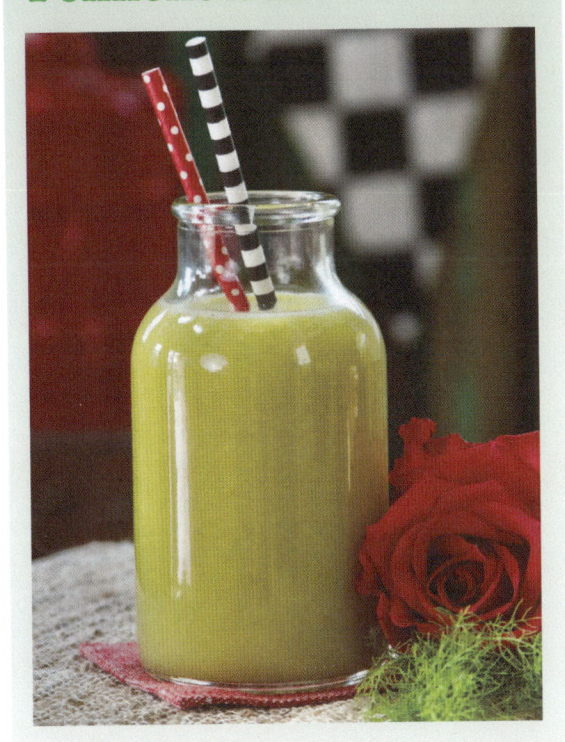

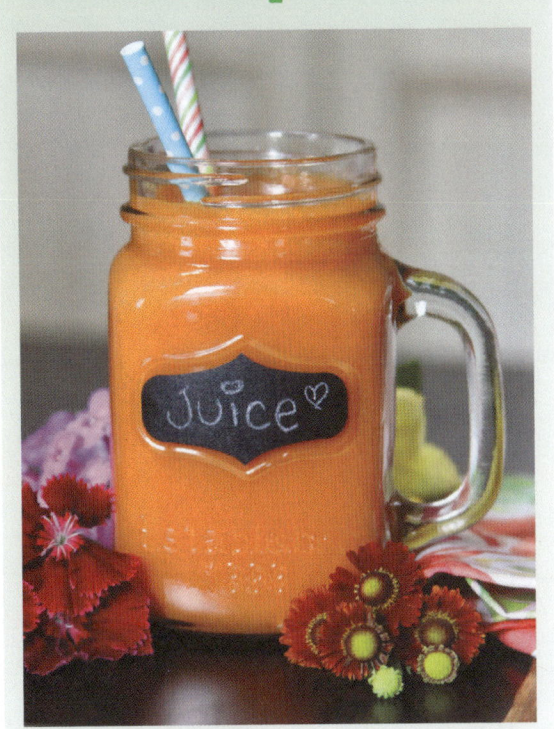

### Ingredients
- 2 apples
- 1 fennel bulb with fronds
- 1 inch ginger
- 1/2 lemon
- 1 orange, peeled
- 10 mint leaves

*Yield: 32 ounces*

# DAY 24
## Lemon Drop

### Ingredients
- 2 apples
- 4 carrots
- 2 inches ginger
- 1 lemon, peeled
- 2 pears
- 1 zucchini

*Yield: 32 ounces*

# DAY 25
## Green Power

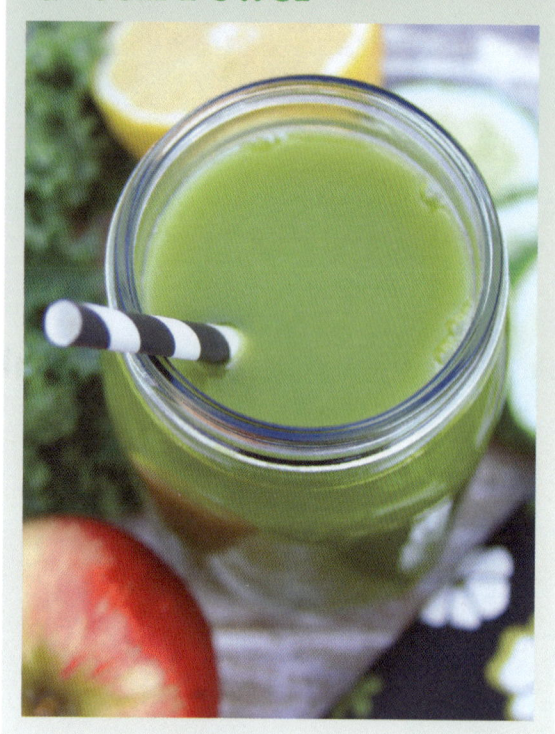

### Ingredients
- 1 avocado
- 1 inch ginger
- 3 kale leaves
- 1/4 lemon
- 1 orange, peeled
- 1 handful parsley
- 1 pear
- 2 1/2 cups pineapple

Yield: 32 ounces

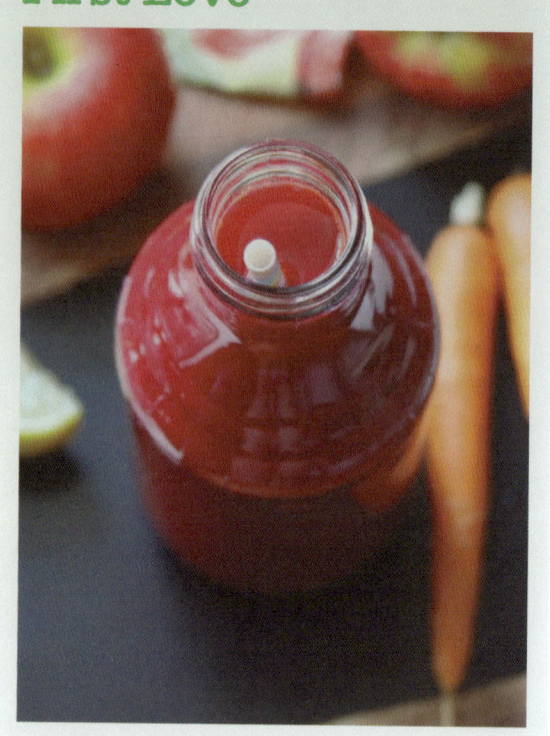

# DAY 26
## First Love

### Ingredients
- 2 apples
- 1 beet
- 4 carrots
- 2 pieces celery
- 1/2 cucumber
- 1/2 inch ginger
- 1/2 lemon
- 1 sweet potato

Yield: 30 ounces

# DAY 27

## Power Aid

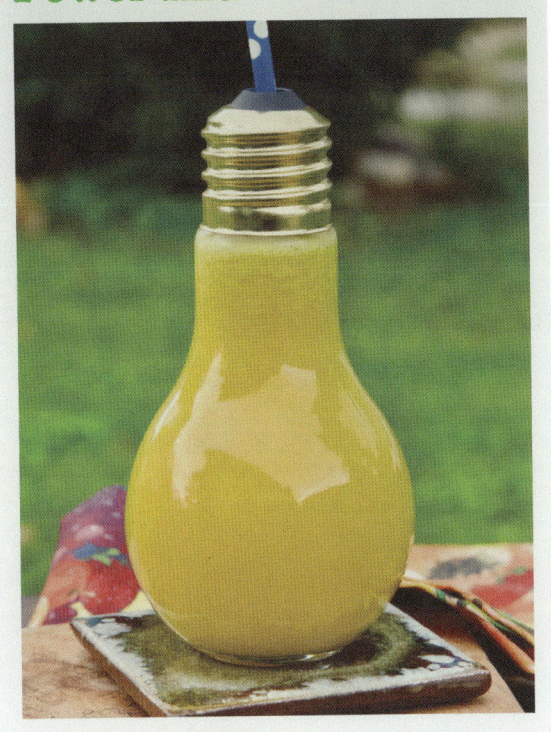

### Ingredients

- 1/2 cucumber
- 2 cups pineapple
- 1/2 lime
- 1 inch ginger

*Yield: 30 ounces*

# DAY 28

## The Game Changer

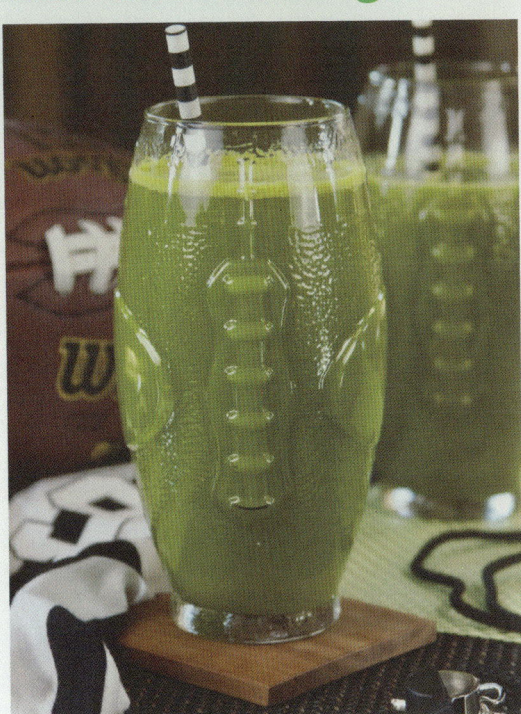

### Ingredients

- 3 cups pineapple
- 1/2 lime
- 1 cucumber
- 2 inches ginger
- 1 orange, peeled
- 3 cups spinach
- 1 dash cayenne

*Yield: 32 ounces*

**Yield**
30 ounces

Pineapple is a good source of vitamin C, potassium and manganese. It may also aid in digestion.

# Day 22: Sweet Adeline

## Ingredients

- 2 apples
- 6 carrots
- 2 pieces celery
- 1 inch ginger
- 2 cups pineapple
- 1 sweet potato

"The ultimate reason for setting goals is to entice you to become the person it takes to achieve them."

— Jim Rohn

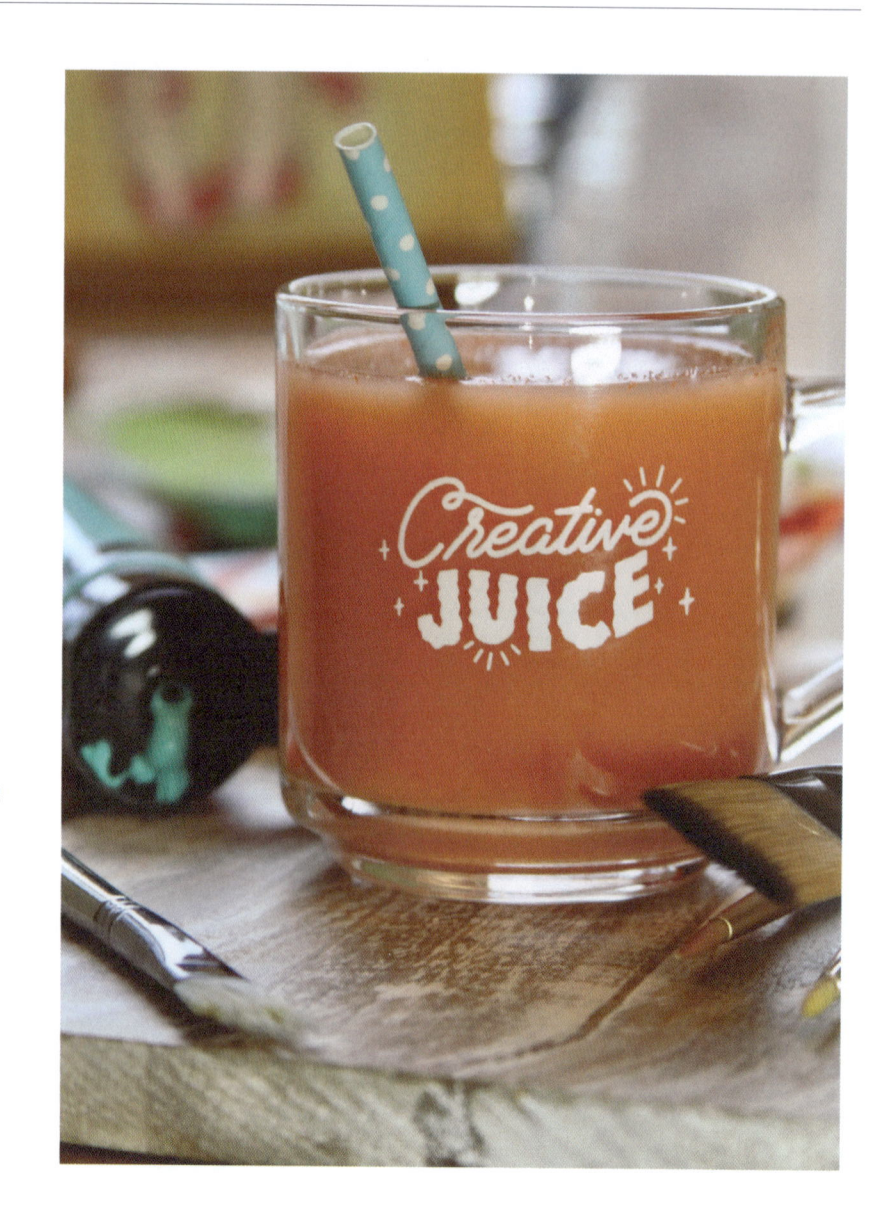

**Yield**
32 ounces

Fennel is good for the skin and bones and may even help lower blood pressure. It has been used for thousands of years as a natural stomach soother, thus aiding in digestion as well.

# Day 23: Fennelicious

## Ingredients

- 2 apples
- 1 fennel bulb with fronds
- 1 inch ginger
- 1/2 lemon
- 1 orange, peeled
- 10 mint leaves

"Instead of living in the shadows of yesterday, live in the light of today and the hope of tomorrow."

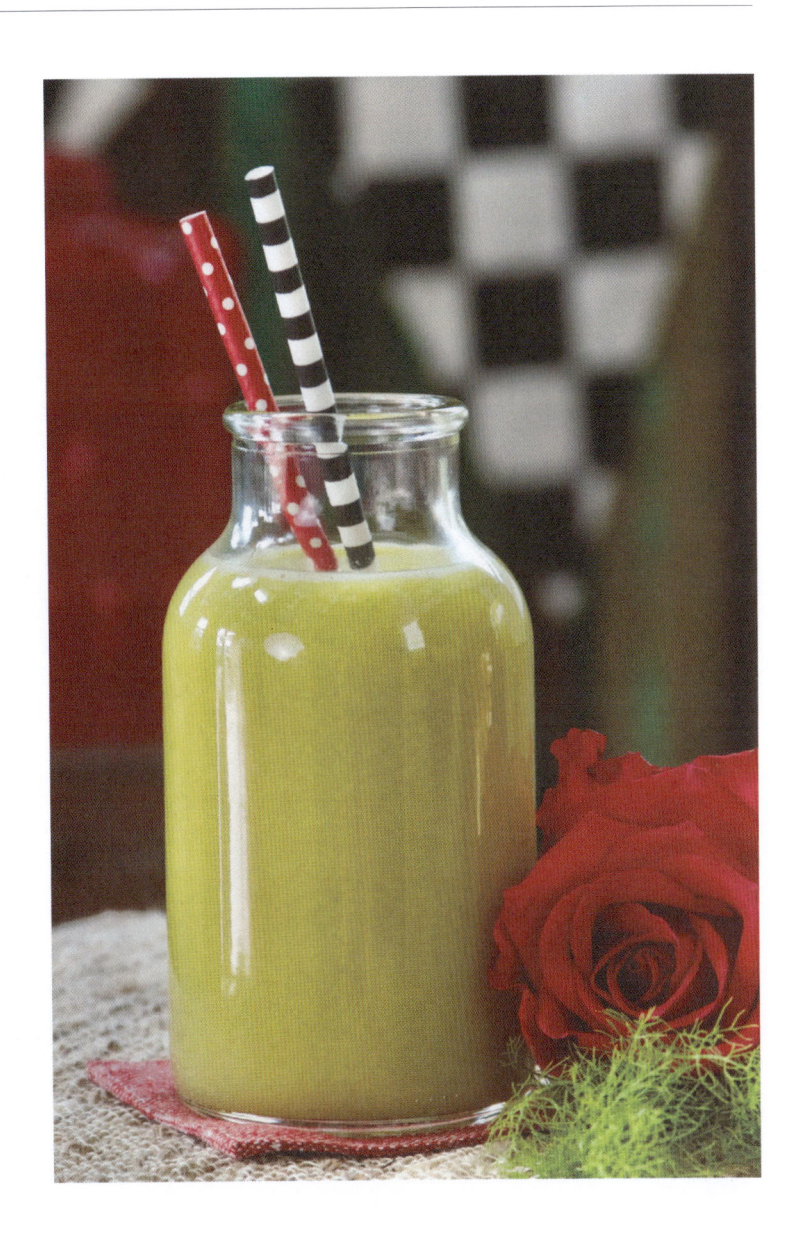

**Yield**
32 ounces

*Pears are a good source of iron and vitamin C. They not only are very alkalizing to the body, but they also add a pleasant flavor to the juice. Pear, lemon and ginger are a match made in heaven.*

# Day 24: Lemon Drop

## Ingredients

- 2 apples
- 4 carrots
- 2 inches ginger
- 1 lemon, peeled
- 2 pears
- 1 zucchini

"Every day is a second chance."

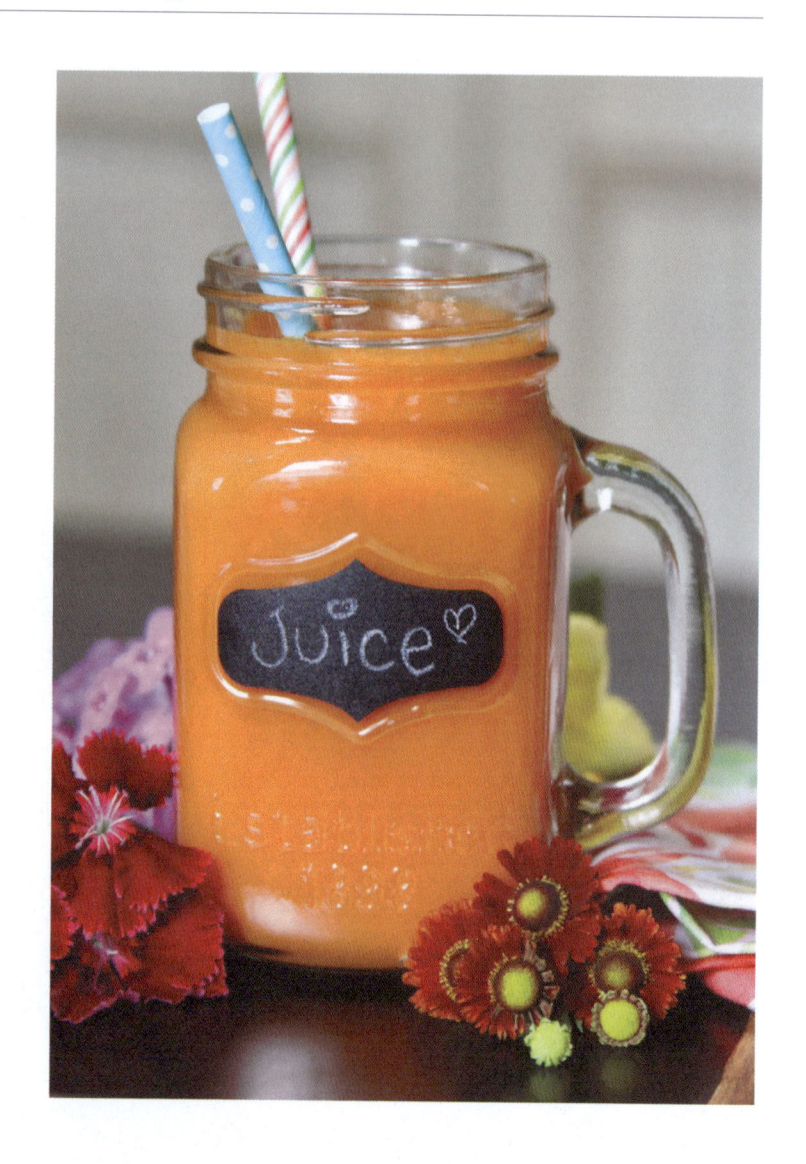

**Yield**
32 ounces

*Have yourself a glass of this plant based power while enjoying every delicious sip!*

# Day 25: Green Power

## Ingredients

- 1 avocado
- 1 inch ginger
- 3 kale leaves
- 1/4 lemon
- 1 orange, peeled
- 1 handful parsley
- 1 pear
- 2 1/2 cups pineapple

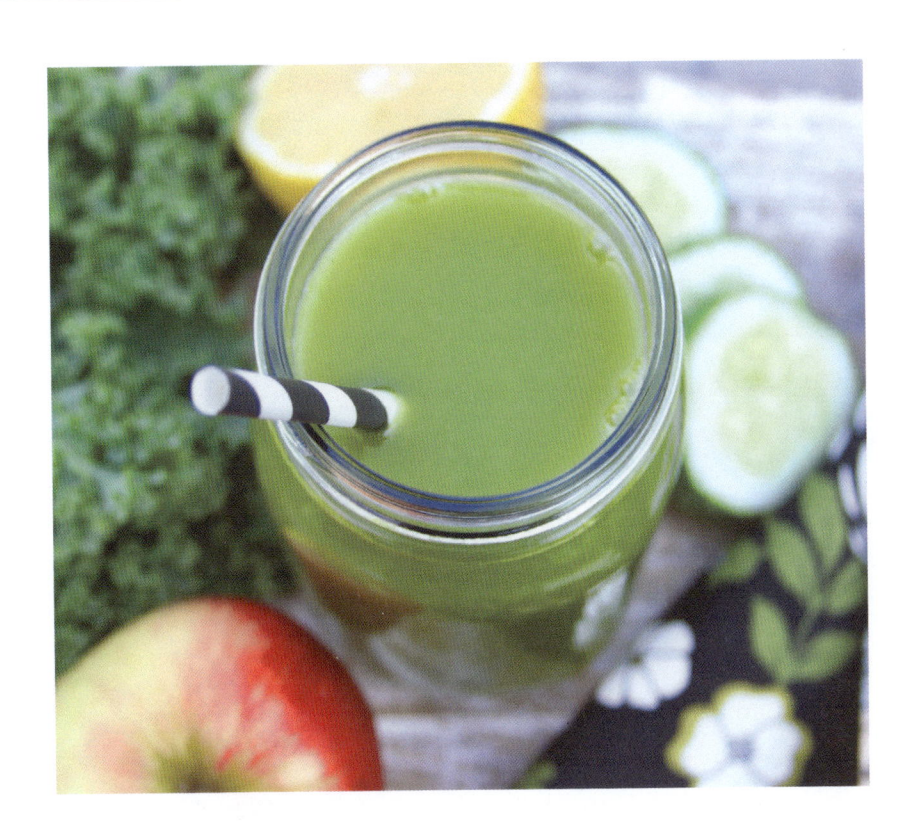

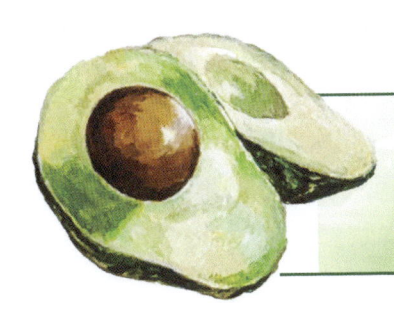

**Directions:** Juice all ingredients together except for the avocado. Blend avocado into the juice with a blender.

**Yield**
30 ounces

*Do you have family members who won't eat fruits and vegetables? My young cousins gave this recipe two thumbs up while standing on a chair (the equivalent of two thumbs up with several exclamation points)!*

# Day 26: First Love

## Ingredients

- 2 apples
- 1 beet
- 4 carrots
- 2 pieces celery
- 1/2 cucumber
- 1/2 inch ginger
- 1/2 lemon
- 1 sweet potato

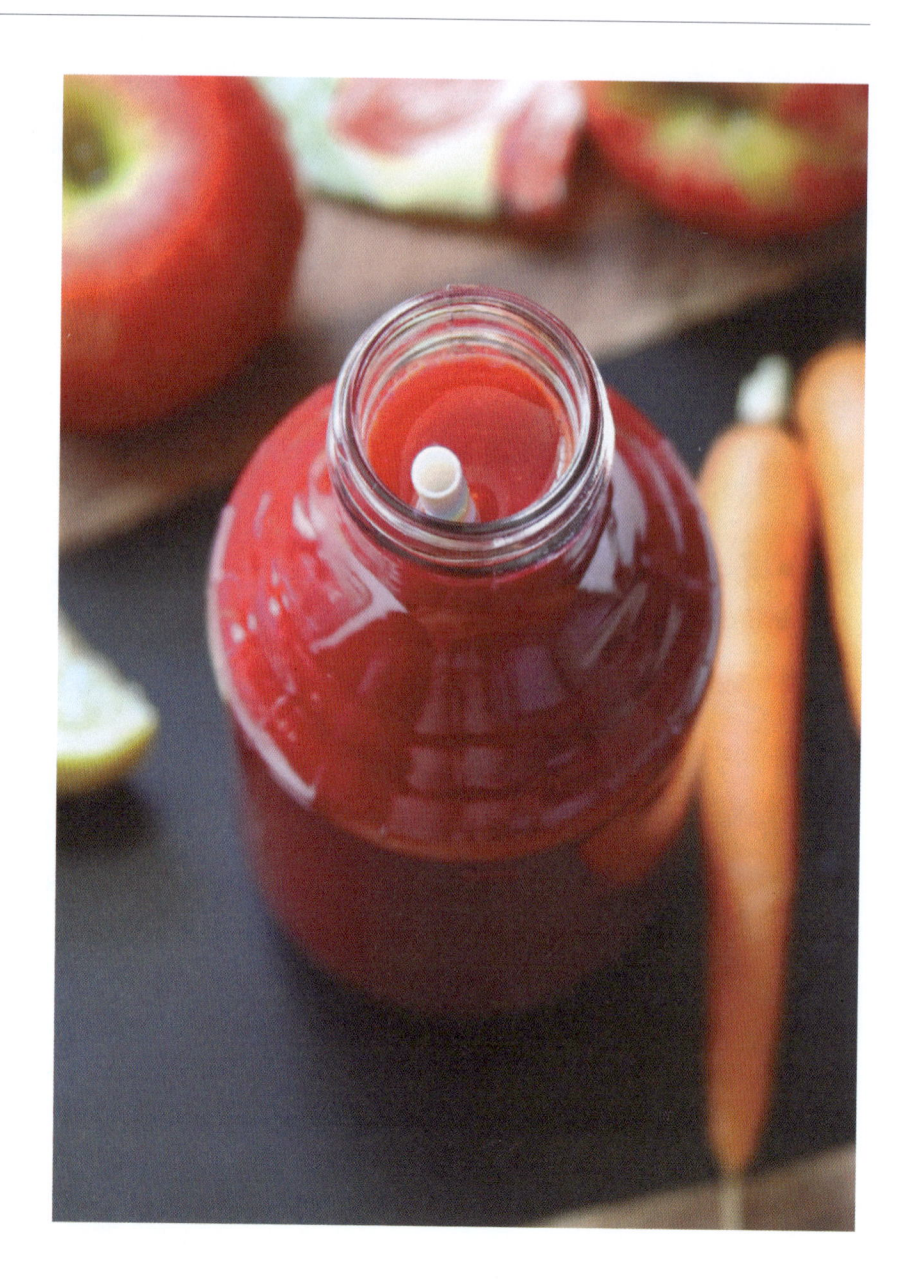

**Yield**
30 ounces

*This juice is not only an excellent source of electrolytes, but it is also very refreshing on a hot day — perfect on ice!*

# Day 27: Power Aid

## Ingredients

- 1/2 cucumber
- 2 cups pineapple
- 1/2 lime
- 1 inch ginger

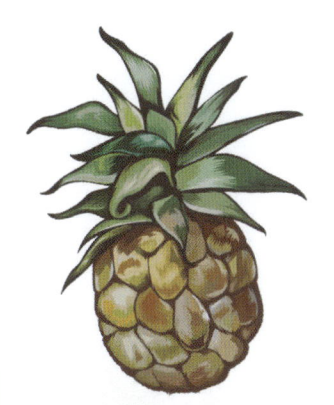

*Turning a pineapple upside down on the counter helps it ripen faster.*

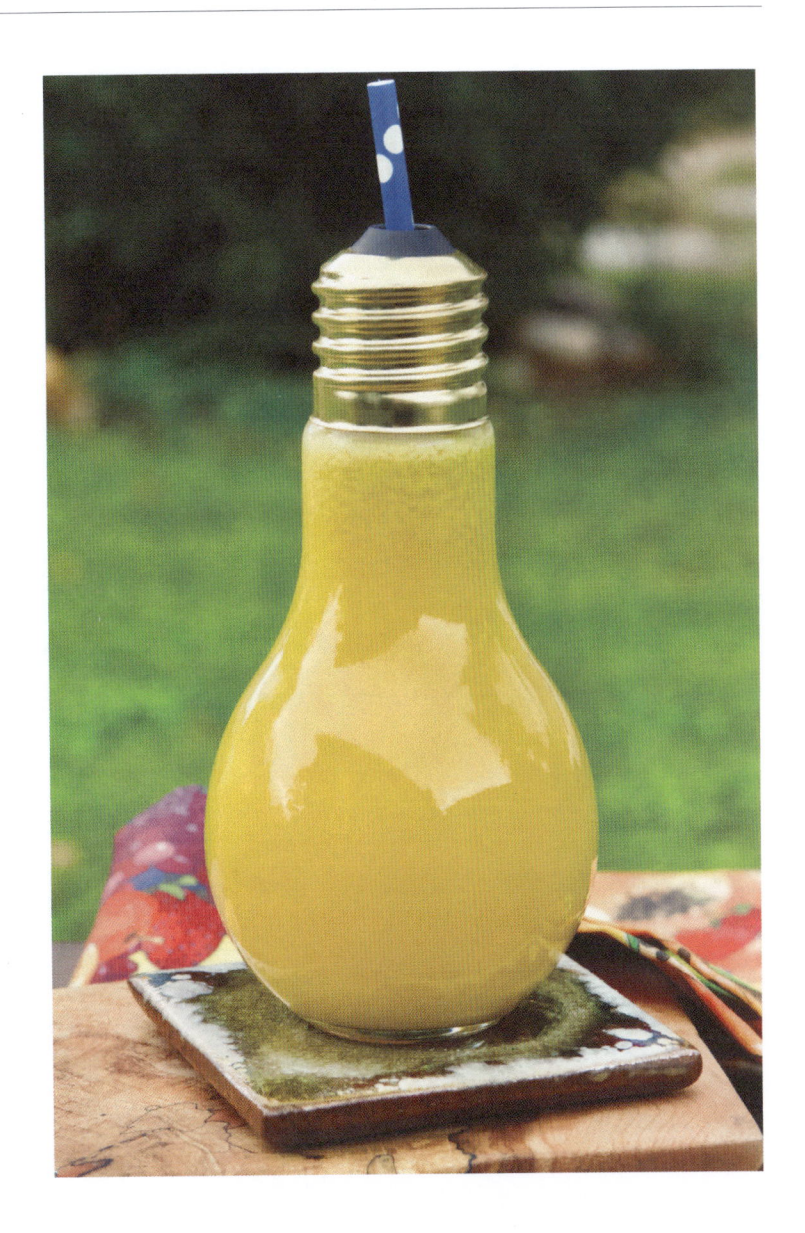

The Challenge: Days 22-28

**Yield**
32 ounces

*Adding cayenne pepper to green juice not only enhances the flavor, but it also adds fat burning properties to the recipe. One of my favorite documentaries is called* **The Game Changers** *and I highly recommend seeing it as it is interesting, informative and inspiring.*

# Day 28: The Game Changer

## Ingredients

- 3 cups pineapple
- 1/2 lime
- 1 cucumber
- 2 inches ginger
- 1 orange, peeled
- 3 cups spinach
- 1 dash cayenne

"Doubt kills more dreams than failure ever will."

— Suzy Kassem

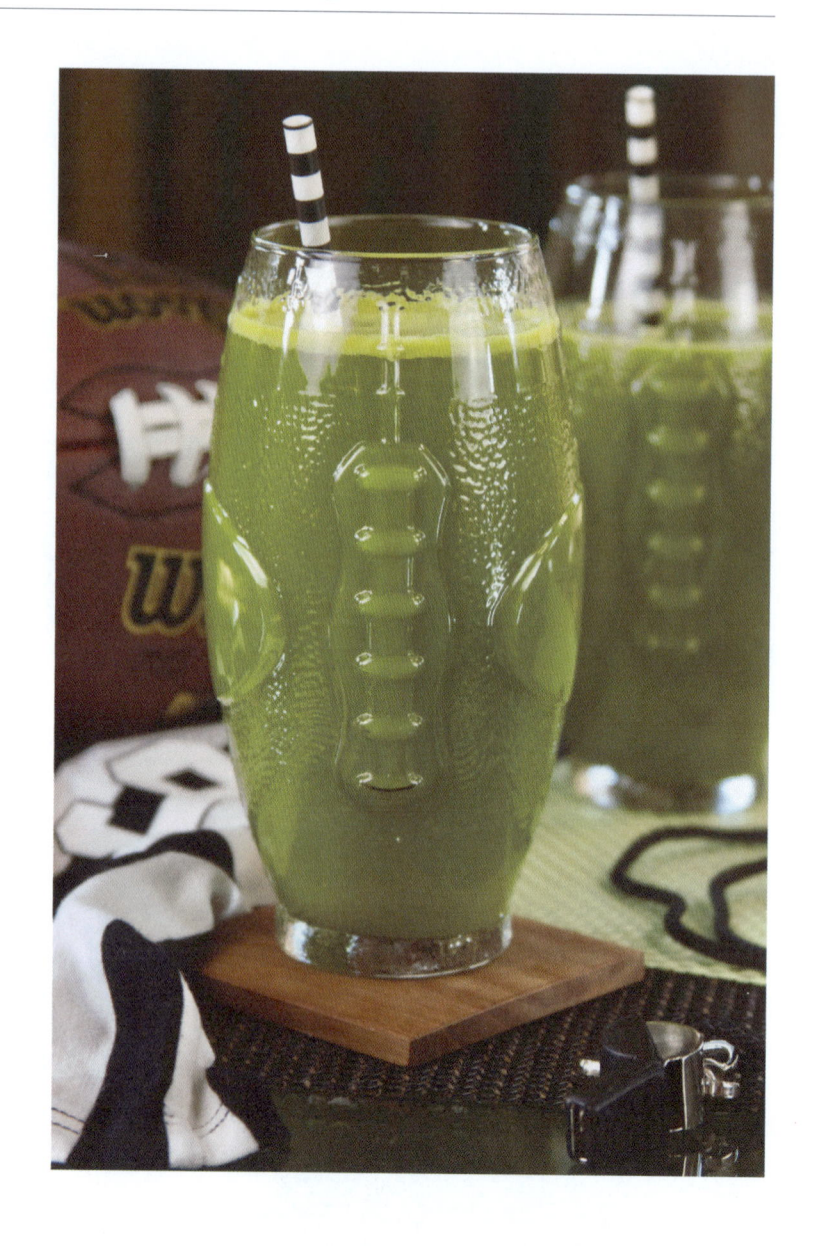

# Days 22-28 Assessment

What were my strongest points this week?

_____
_____
_____

Did I juice or have juice every day of the challenge? _____

What was my favorite recipe? _____

Were there any unexpected obstacles? If so, how did I handle them with regards to juicing?

_____
_____
_____

Is there anything I can do to prepare for next week to make it even better?

_____
_____
_____

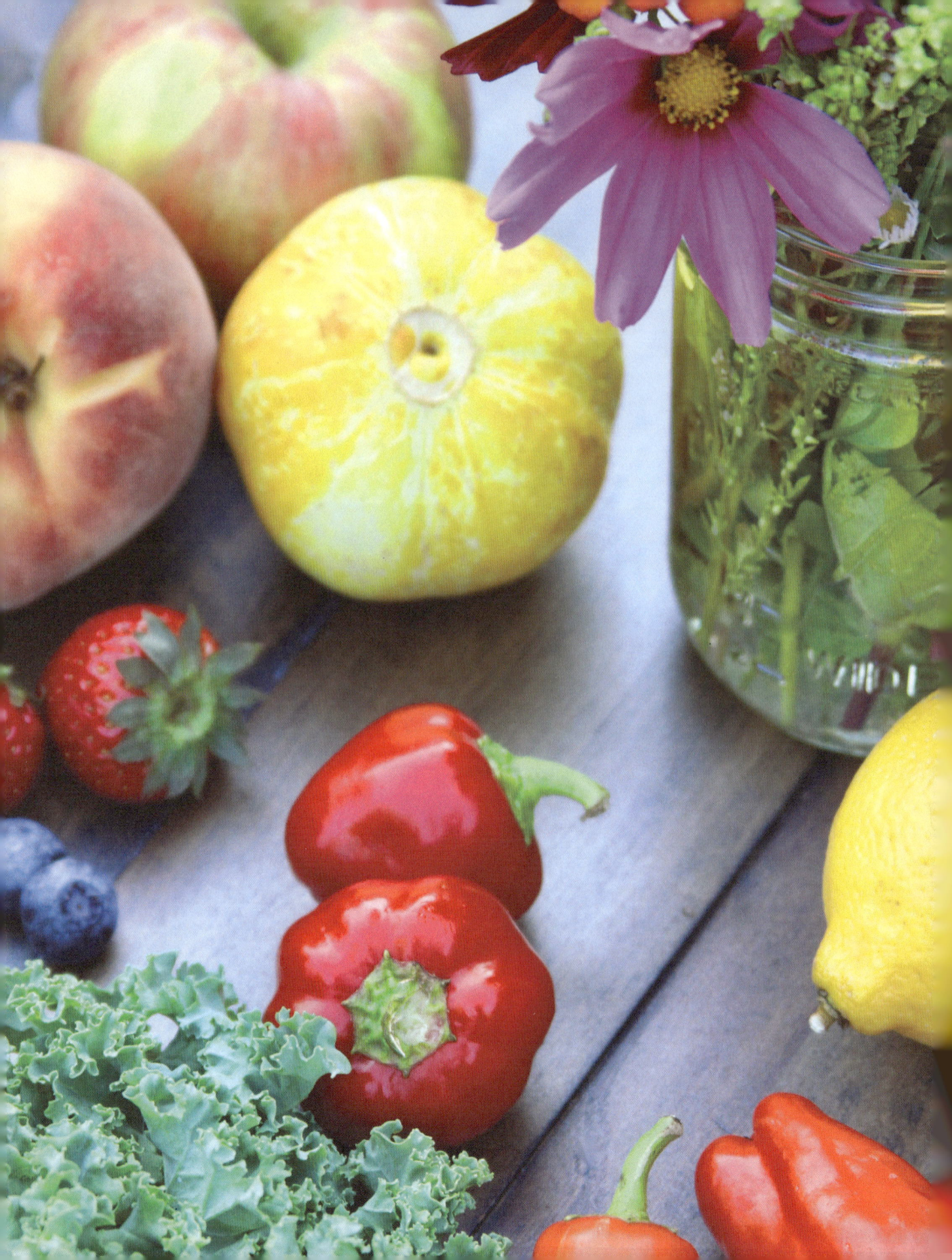

# Days 29-30 Shopping List

**You've got this!** You're in the final stretch! May you finish strong, and may the last two days be your best two days!

## Vegetables

- ☐ 1 beet
- ☐ 6 carrots
- ☐ 5 pieces celery
- ☐ 2 cucumbers
- ☐ 2 cups spinach

## Herbs & Spices

- ☐ 2 inches ginger
- ☐ 1 bunch parsley

## Fruits

- ☐ 4 apples
- ☐ 1 lemon
- ☐ 1 lime
- ☐ 1 orange

The Challenge: Days 29-30

# DAY 29

## Dr. Oz's Green Drink

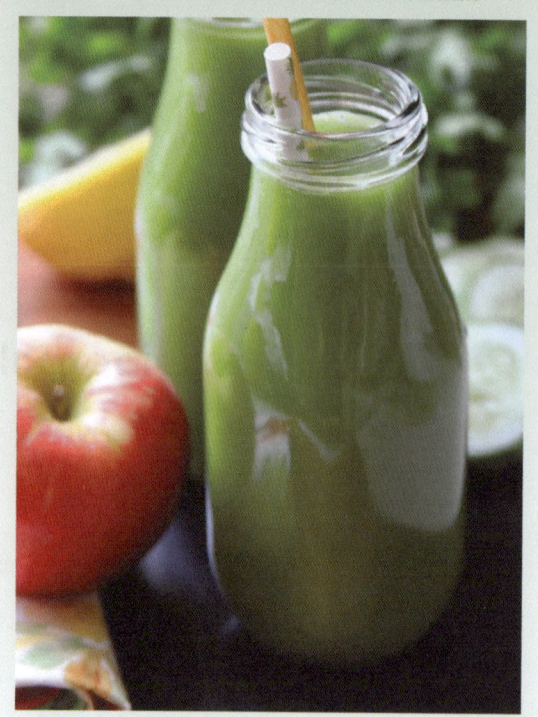

### Ingredients

- 2 apples
- 3 celery
- 1 cucumber
- 1 inch ginger
- 1/2 lemon
- 1 lime
- 1 handful parsley
- 2 cups spinach

*Yield: 32 ounces*

# DAY 30

## Candy Crush

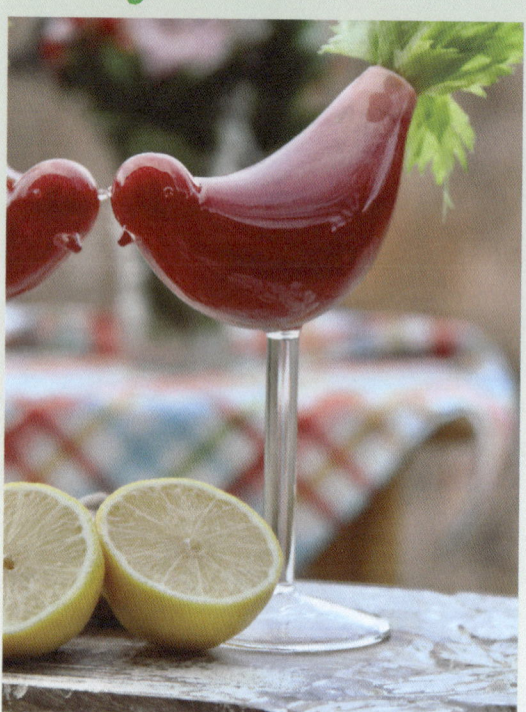

### Ingredients

- 2 apples
- 1 beet
- 6 carrots
- 2 celery
- 1/2 cucumber
- 1 inch of ginger
- 1 orange, peeled
- 1/2 lemon

*Yield: 32 ounces*

**Yield**
32 ounces

*This recipe is bursting with vitamins, minerals and enzymes. It has liver and kidney cleansing properties and works well as a meal replacement.*

# Day 29: Dr. Oz's Green Drink

## Ingredients

- 2 apples
- 3 celery
- 1 cucumber
- 1 inch ginger
- 1/2 lemon
- 1 lime
- 1 handful parsley
- 2 cups spinach

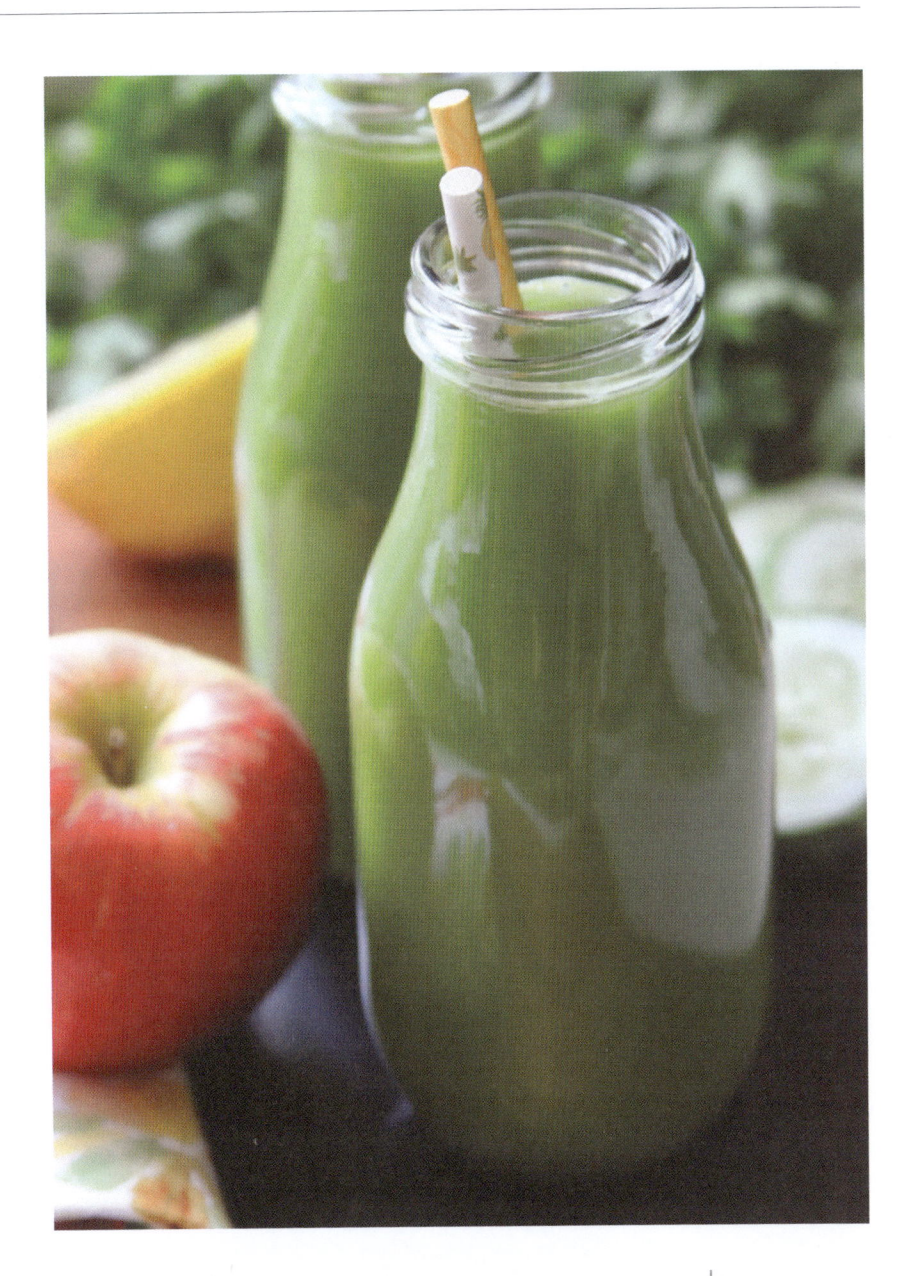

The Challenge: Days 29-30

**Yield**
32 ounces

*Here we are on the final day of this challenge! I hope you have found it to be rewarding in every way possible and are feeling better than ever!*

# Day 30: Candy Crush

## Ingredients

- 2 apples
- 1 beet
- 6 carrots
- 2 celery
- 1/2 cucumber
- 1 inch of ginger
- 1 orange, peeled
- 1/2 lemon

"A goal properly set is halfway reached."

— Zig Ziglar

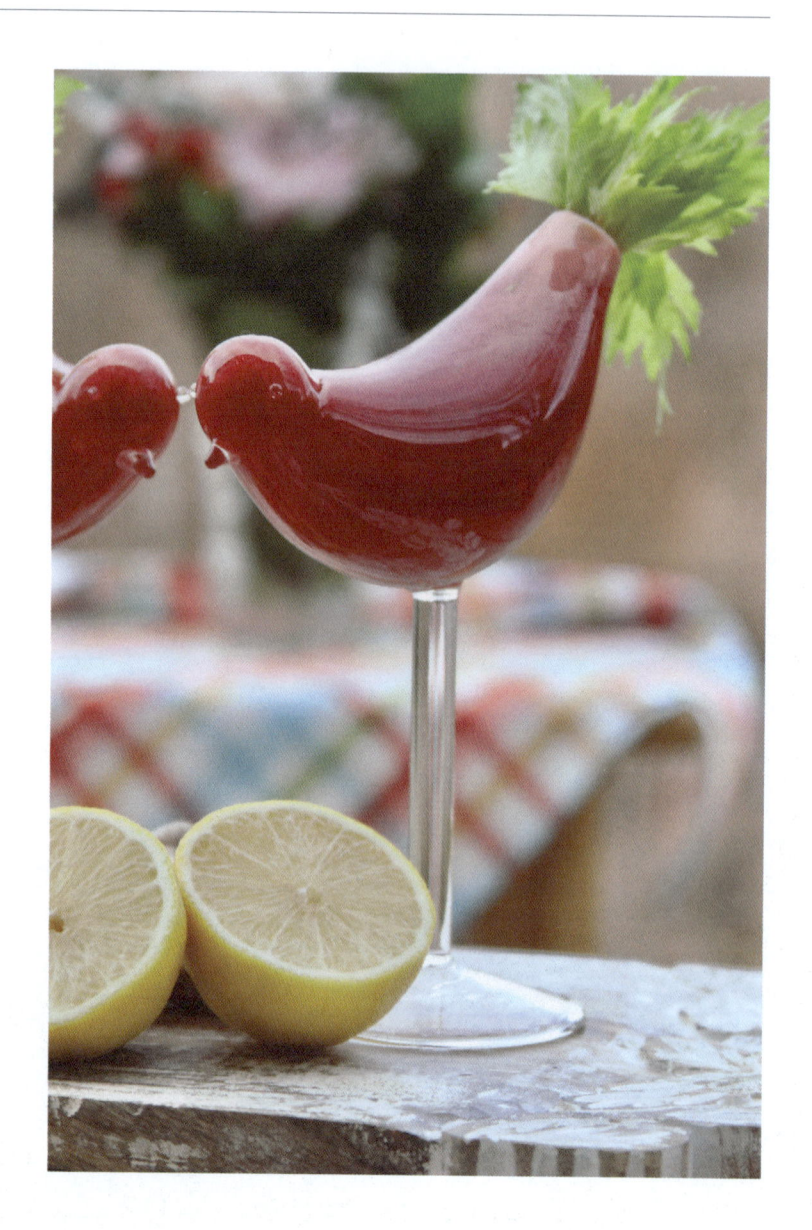

# Final Assessment

What were my strongest points over the entire 30 days?
_____
_____
_____

Did I juice or have juice every day of the challenge? _____

What was my all-time favorite recipe? _____

What were my biggest obstacles? How did I handle them with regards to juicing?
_____
_____
_____

What would I like to do next to maintain the habit of juicing? (Take the challenge again, do a juice cleanse, have a meeting with my partner or friends about the next step to take?)
_____
_____
_____

*Congratulations on completing your 30 days of juicing! Hope you are feeling stronger, healthier and more vibrant than you were last month.*

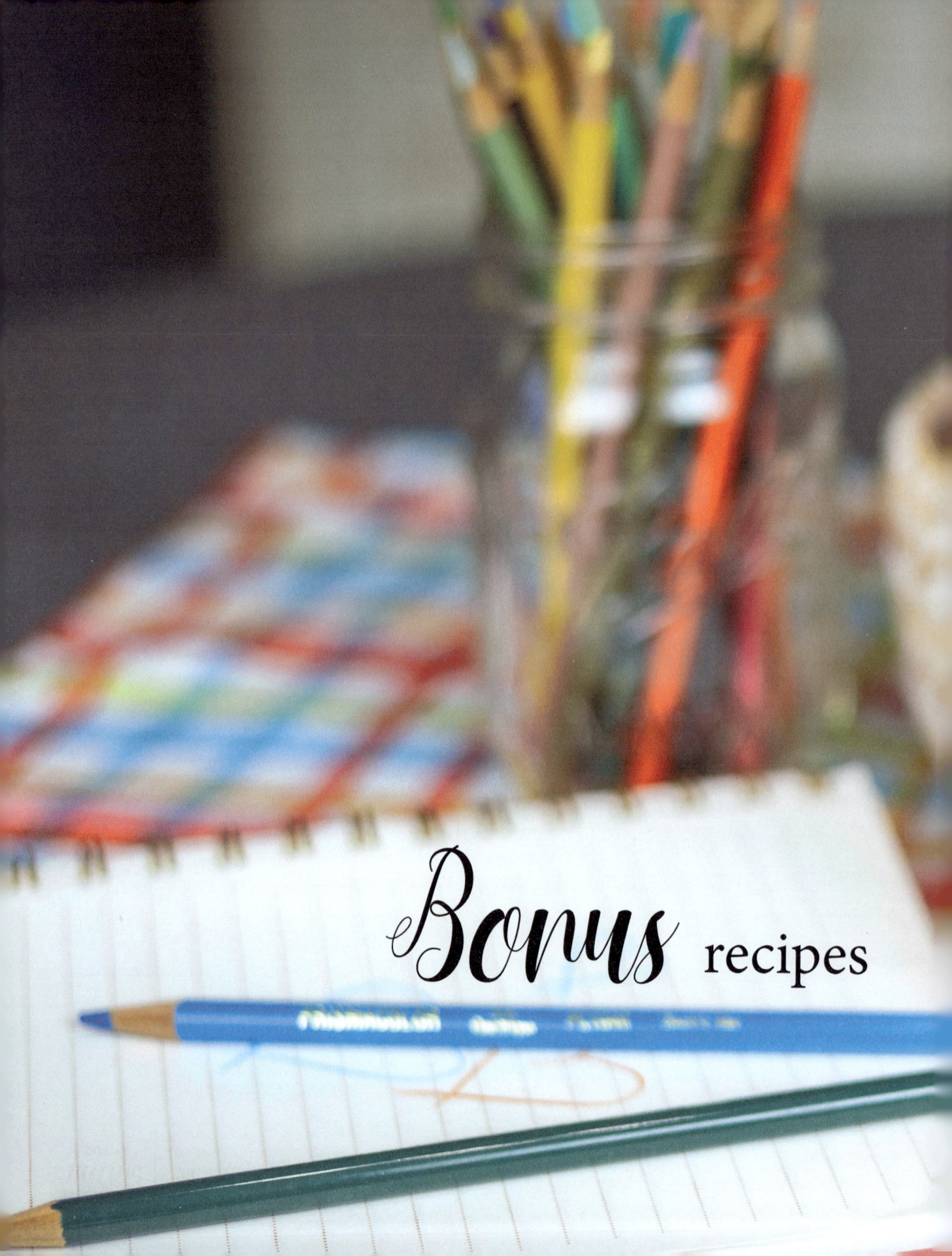

# Bonus recipes

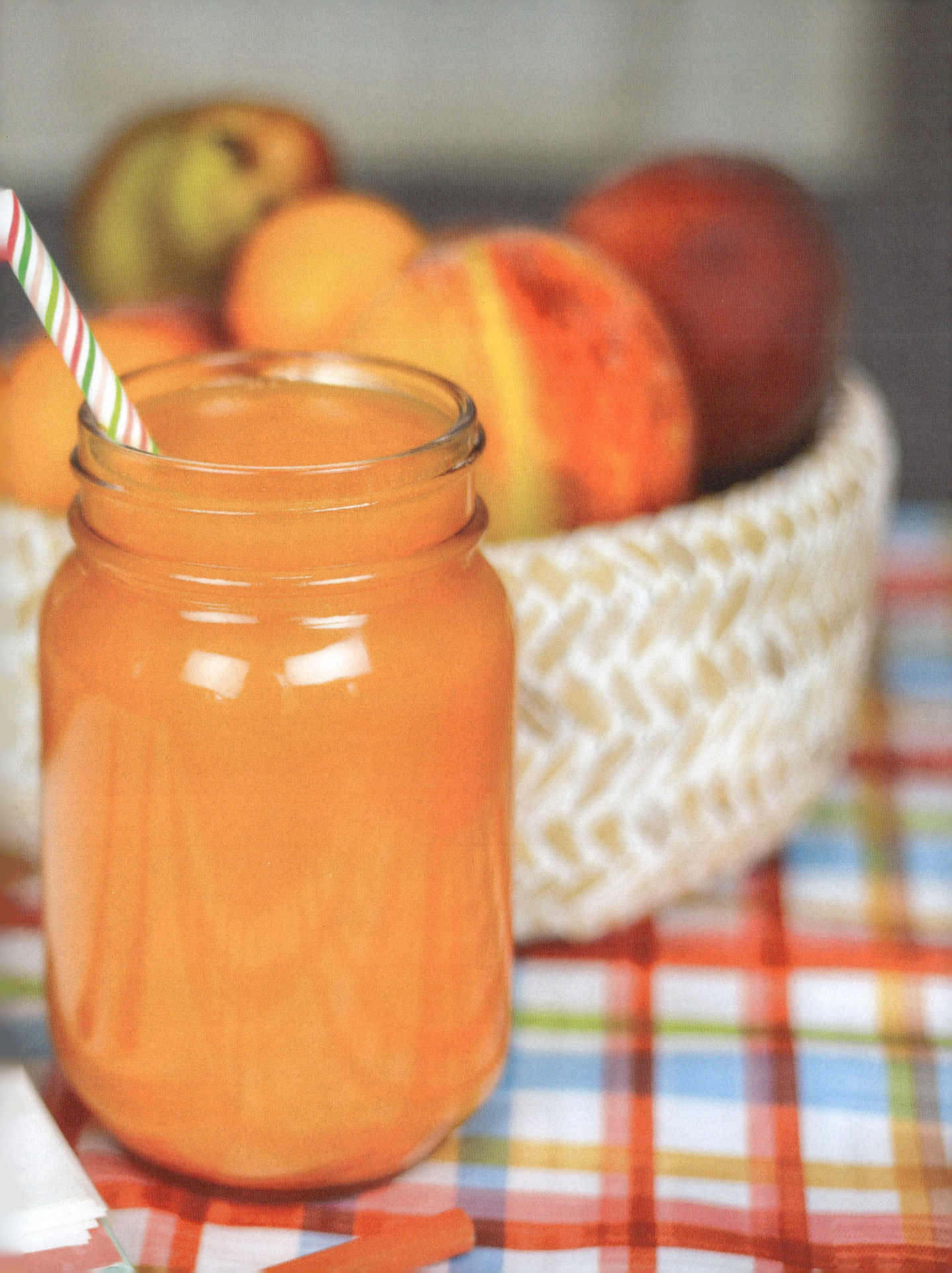

# Bonus Recipes

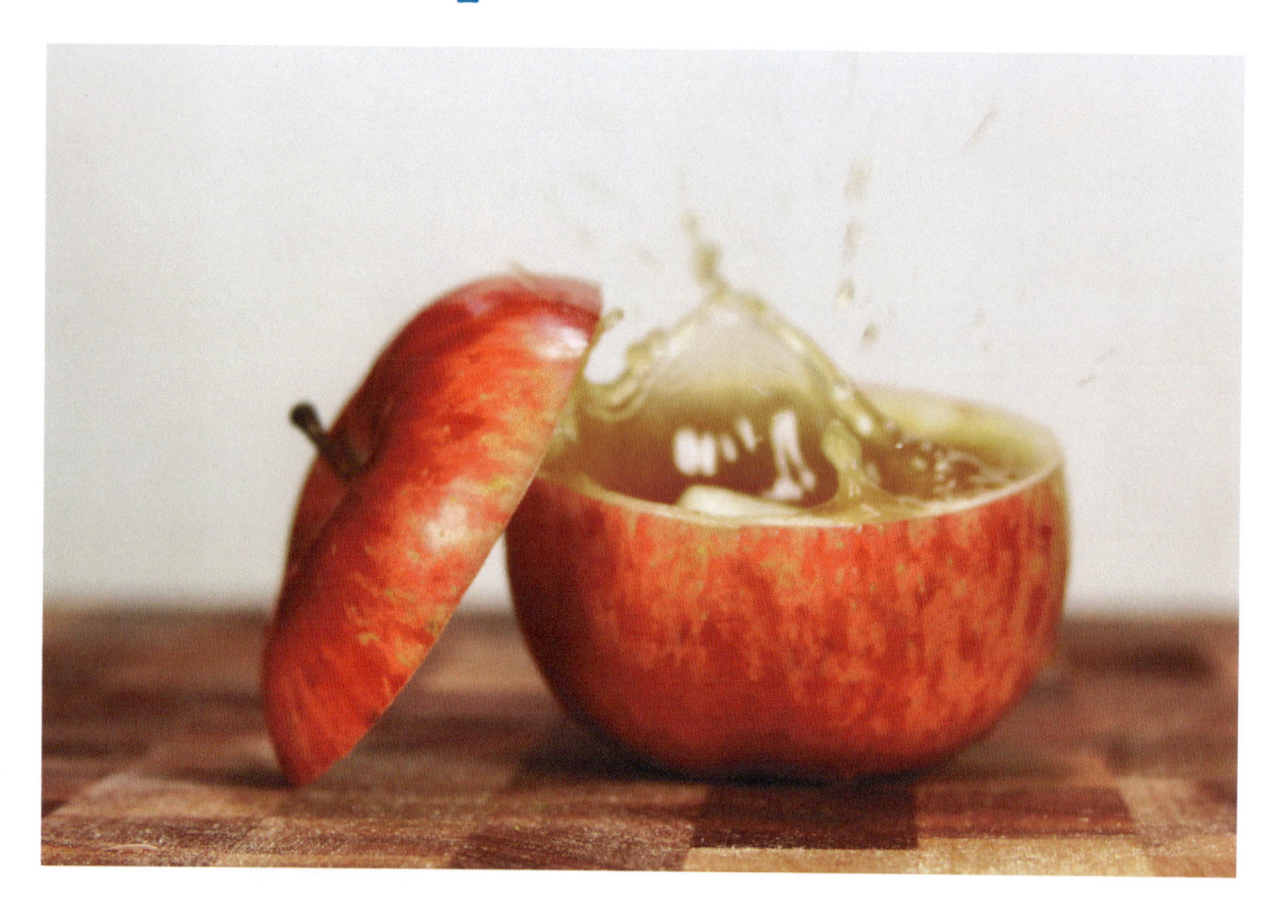

### Peachy Keen
- 3 fresh basil leaves
- 14 carrots
- 1/2 lemon
- 5 peaches

Yield: 32 ounces

### Lemon Essence
- 1 apple
- 8 carrots
- 1 lemon
- 1 inch ginger

Yield: 26 ounces

### High Five!
- 2 apples
- 1 beet
- 1/2 cucumber
- 1/4 lemon
- 3 cups pineapple

Yield: 28 ounces

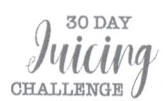

## Green Vibes

- 1 apple
- 4 pieces celery
- 1 1/2 inches ginger
- 1 lemon
- 2 handfuls spinach
- 1/2 zucchini

Yield: 18 ounces

## Morning Bliss

- 2 apples
- 5 carrots
- 2 pieces celery
- 2 inches ginger
- 1/2 lemon
- 1 orange, peeled
- 1 sweet potato
- 1 piece turmeric

Yield: 30 ounces

## Blue Lagoon Lemonade

- 1 cup blueberries
- 1 cup green or white tea
- 1 inch ginger
- 1 teaspoon honey
- 1/2 lemon
- 2 cups pineapple
- 1 cup strawberries

Yield: 30 ounces

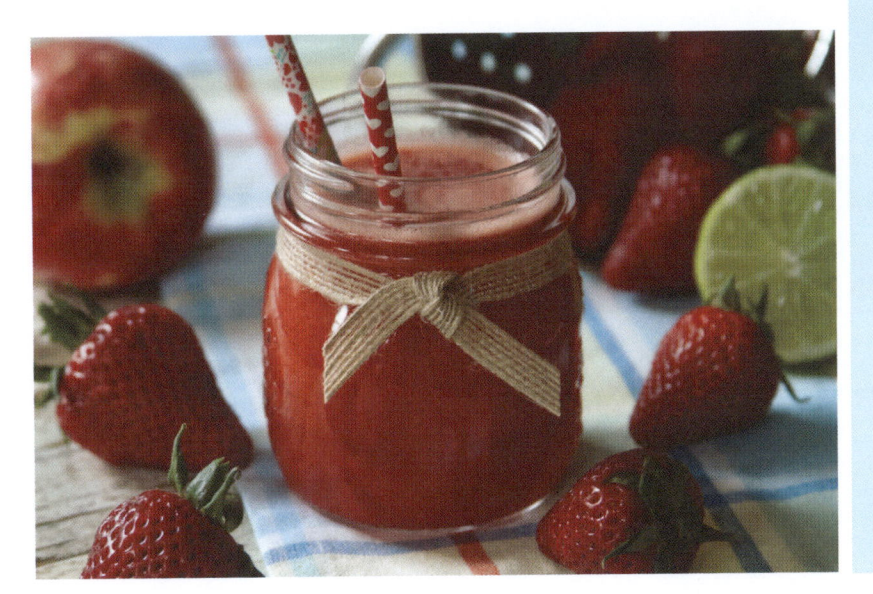

Directions

1. Make one cup of tea as directed.
2. Add honey and cool.
3. Juice the other ingredients
4. Stir ingredients together and enjoy. (Goes great on ice!)

Bonus Recipes

## Fresh Start 2

- 2 apples
- 8 carrots
- 2 pieces celery

Yield: 16 ounces

## The Liver Scrubber

- 1 apple
- 1 beet
- 4 carrots
- 1 piece celery
- 1 inch ginger

Yield: 16 ounces

## Watermelon Sugar

- 1 apple
- 1/4 lime
- 7 mint leaves
- 1/2 cup strawberries
- 2 cups watermelon

Yield: 22 ounces

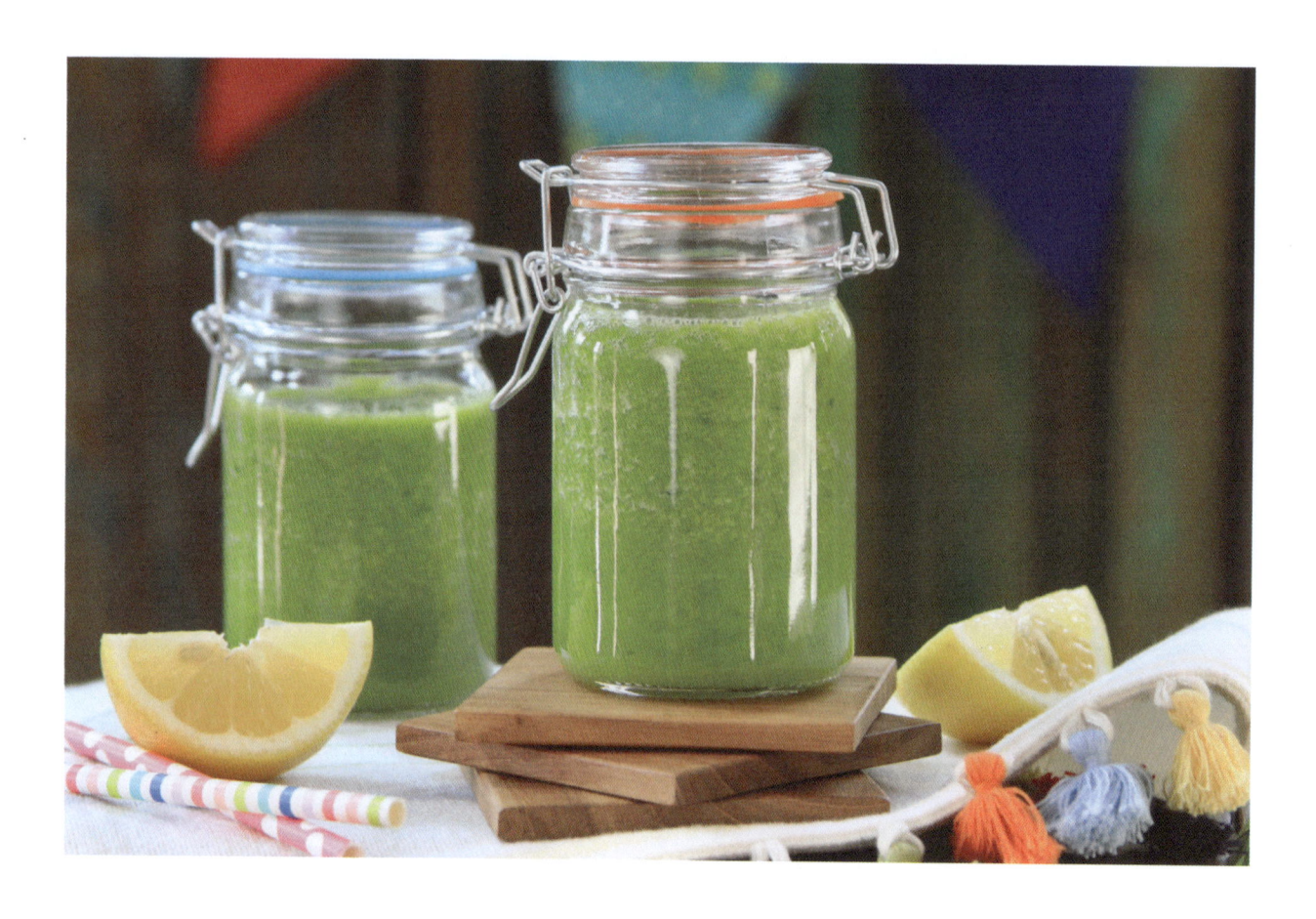

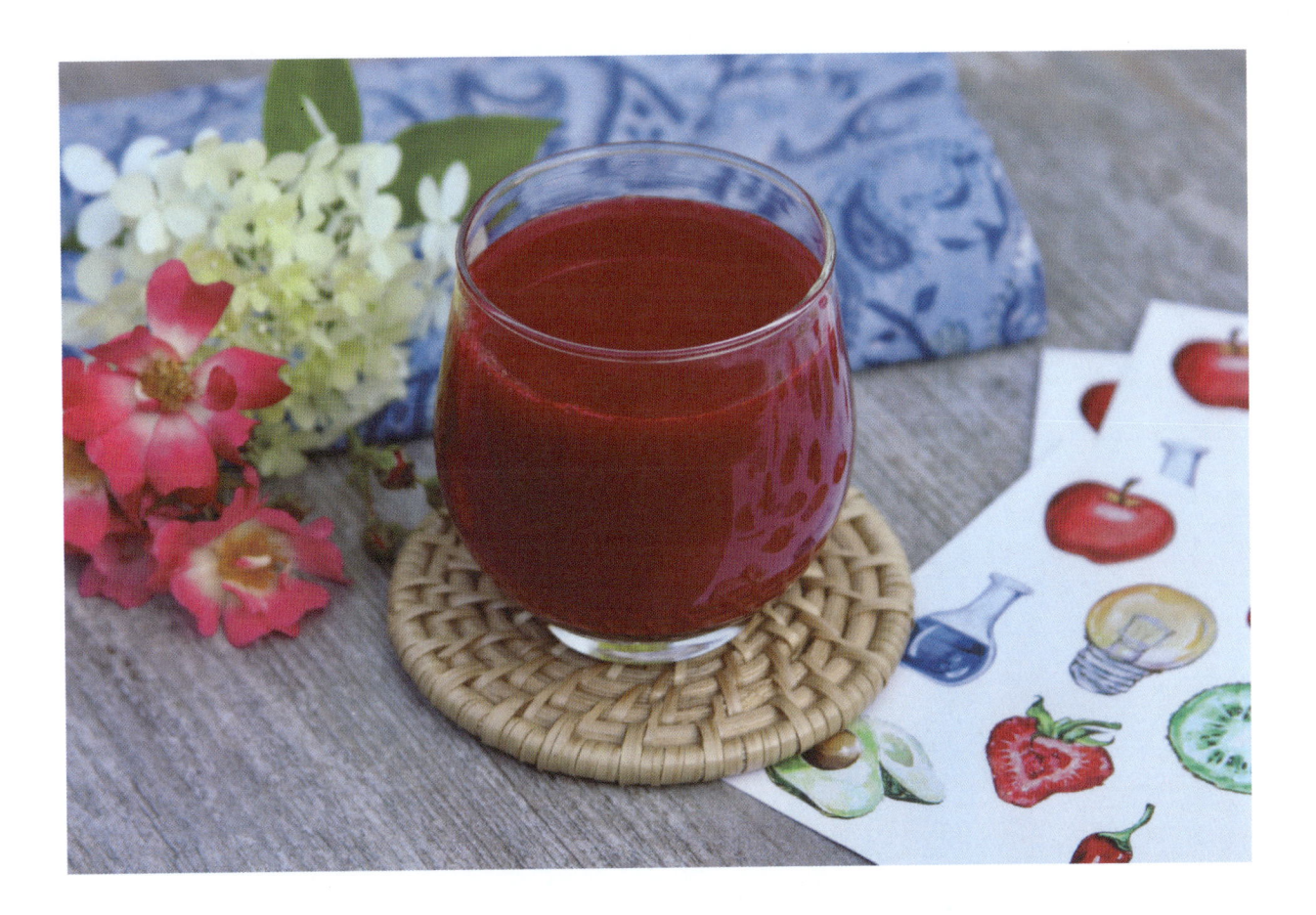

## Sweet Potato Pie

- 2 apples
- 6 carrots
- 1 sweet potato
- 1 dash cinnamon

*Yield: 18 ounces*

## Kale'd It

- 3 basil leaves
- 1 handful Italian parsley
- 5 kale leaves
- 1 orange
- 1 pear
- 1 zucchini

*Yield: 20 ounces*

## Berry A Pealing

- 2 apples
- 1/2 lime
- 3 cups strawberries

*Yield: 20 ounces*

Bonus Recipes

# Making Your Nut Milk Delicious!

- Use raw or pasteurized nuts.
- You need a slow or masticating juicer to make almond or other nut milks.
- Soak the nuts for at least 4 hours to overnight.
- Drain the soak water and discard. It contains enzyme inhibitors that may give some people an upset stomach.
- Make sure you have a combination of both water and nuts when pouring them through the juicer, or the nuts will go straight into the pulp without making milk.
- I prefer using Medjool dates to sweeten my almond milk, and I run them through the juicer with the water and nuts.
- Remember to remove the pits from the dates before running them through the juicer.
- You don't have to take the skins off of the almonds before you juice them, but I do because the consistency of the milk is smoother than when the skins remain. It also makes for a smoother pulp if you are using it in cake or cookies.
- I add Himalayan salt to my nut milks, not only for the minerals, but because I have noticed the milk stays fresher longer.
- For a smoother nut milk, strain with a fine mesh strainer or nut milk bag.
- The nut milk pulp can be frozen and used at a later time.

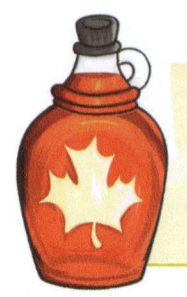

*Running the almond pulp through the juicer a second time with two additional cups of water increases the yield by almost a quart.*

**Yield**
2 quarts

*This almond milk has been kitchen tested to perfection and is a much requested favorite of family and friends.*

# Almond Pecan Milk

## Ingredients

- 1 cup almonds
- 1 cup pecans
- 4-5 pitted Medjool dates
- 1-2 inches vanilla bean
- Himalayan salt to taste
- 4-5 cups purified water

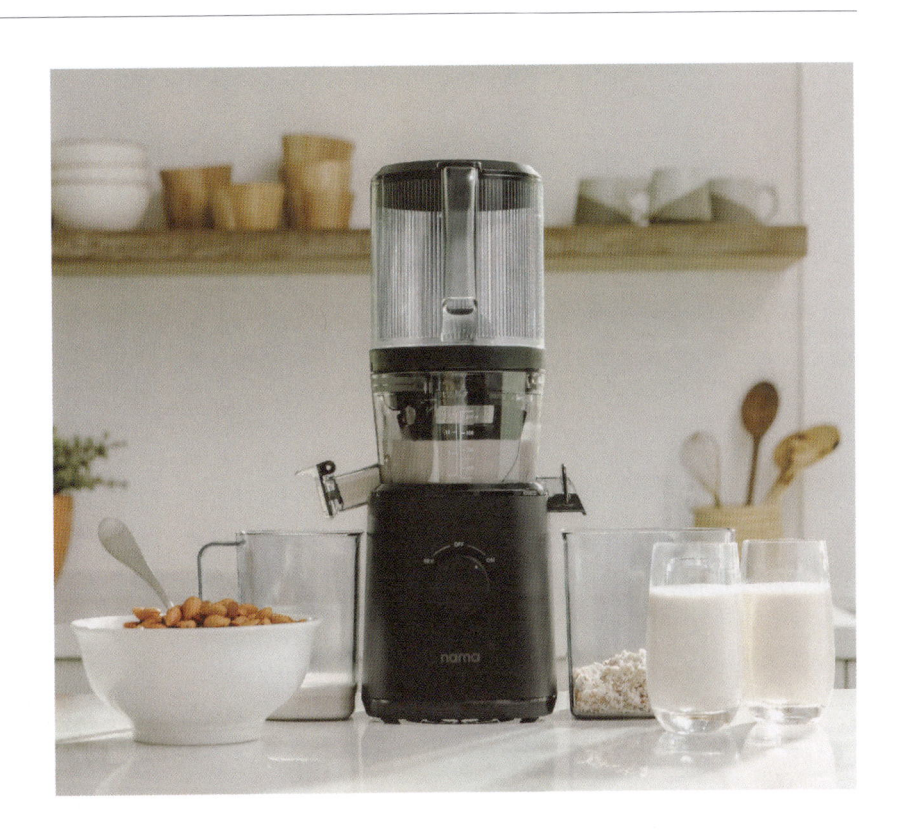

## Directions

1. Soak the almonds and pecans overnight.
2. Drain the soak water, and add the 4-5 cups of purified water to the almonds, pecans, dates and vanilla bean.
3. Juice all ingredients together at the same time, being sure the water is included with the almonds and pecans.
4. Strain milk with a fine mesh strainer and add salt.
5. Drink immediately, or store in mason jars in the refrigerator until ready to use. (Usually lasts at least 72 hours.)

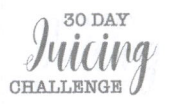

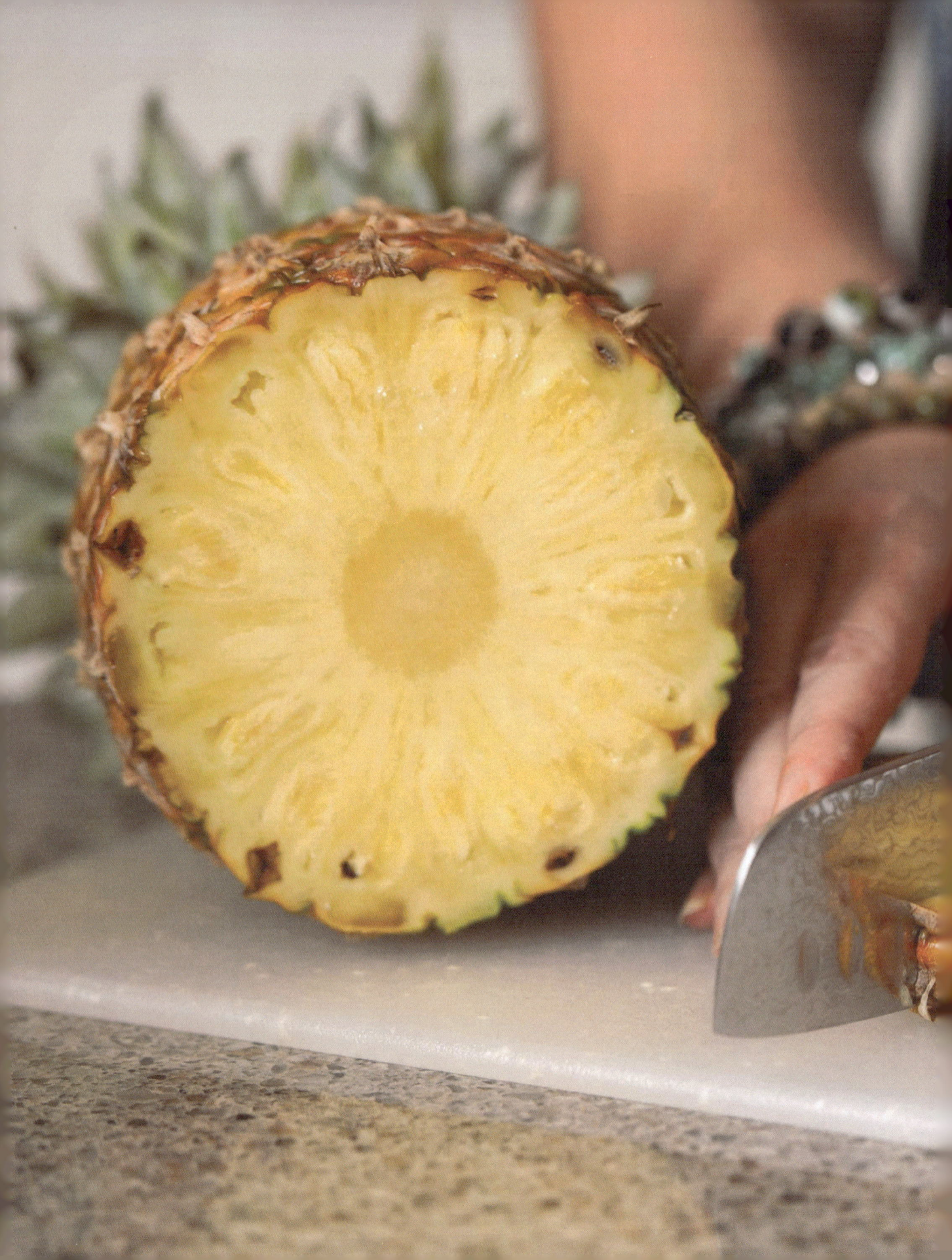

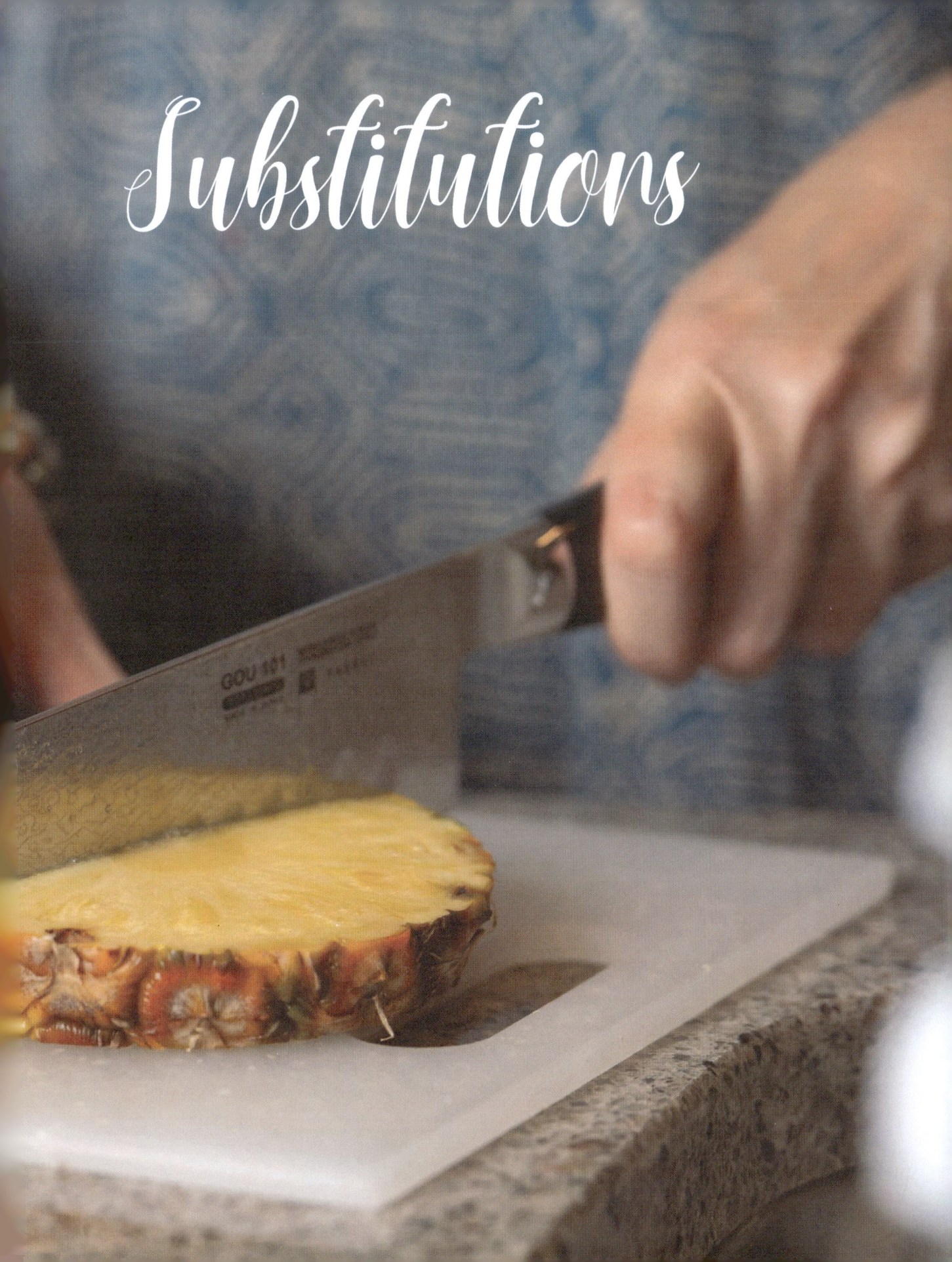

# Substitutions

Are you ready to make a juice and find you are missing an ingredient? Perhaps you have an allergy to a certain fruit or vegetable. Maybe you can't find what you're looking for at the grocery store or farmer's market. Here are some ideas for substitutions, although you may want to look at the other ingredients in your juice as you make your decision!

## A

**Almond milk** — Cashew milk, coconut milk, other nut milks
**Apple** — Any variety, pear, grapes (any type), cherries, blackberries, blueberries
**Arugula (Rocket)** — Spinach, kale, watercress
**Avocado** — Roasted veggies (squash, mushroom, eggplant)

## B

**Banana** — Avocado, yogurt, coconut milk, other nut milks
**Basil** — Parsley, cilantro, mint
**Beets (Beetroot)** — Red cabbage, tomato, radish, golden beets
**Blueberries** — Blackberries, strawberries, raspberries, cherries
**Bok choy** — Kale, beet greens, dandelion greens, arugula
**Broccoli stalk** — Celery, cucumber, cauliflower
**Broccoli** — Cauliflower, green cabbage, kale, chard
**Butternut squash** — Pumpkin, carrot, sweet potato, any winter squash

## C

**Cantaloupe** — Mango, papaya, peach, honeydew melon
**Carrots** — Sweet potato, winter squash, pumpkin, parsnip
**Celery** — Cucumber, zucchini, jicama, romaine lettuce

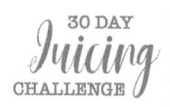

**Cherries** — Raspberries, strawberries, blackberries
**Chives** — Scallions, green onion
**Cilantro** — Basil, Italian parsley, curly parsley
**Coconut milk** — Yogurt, water, any nut milk
**Coconut water** — Water, diluted fresh juice, sometimes cucumber
**Collard greens** — Mustard greens, kale, beet greens, dandelion greens, spinach
**Cranberries** — Cherries, raspberries, strawberries
**Cucumber** — Celery, zucchini, summer squash

## D

**Dandelion green** — Kale, mustard or collard greens, beet greens, chard, spinach, romaine
**Dates** — Honey, pure maple syrup

## F

**Fennel** — Celery, kohlrabi, endive

## G

**Garlic** — Shallot, green onion
**Ginger** — Lemon
**Grapefruit** — Clementine, orange, tangerine, blood orange, cara cara orange
**Green beans** — Asparagus, kale
**Green cabbage** — Red/purple cabbage, kale, arugula, chard
**Green peppers (capsicum)** — Red or yellow peppers
**Green tea** — White tea, oolong tea, black tea, silver needle tea

## H

**Honey** — Dates, pure maple syrup, coconut sugar
**Honeydew (melon)** — Green grapes, cantaloupe, apple, watermelon

## J

**Jalapeño (chili pepper)** — Any other hot pepper, green bell pepper

## K

**Kale** — Arugula, spinach, Swiss chard, green cabbage, mustard/collard/beet/turnip greens, beet greens, romaine
**Kiwi** — Mango, orange, tangerine, lime

## L

**Lemon** — Lime, ginger
**Lime** — Lemon, orange, ginger

## M

**Mango** — Papaya, kiwi
**Maple syrup** — Honey, agave
**Mint** — Ginger, basil

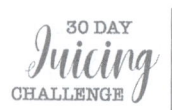

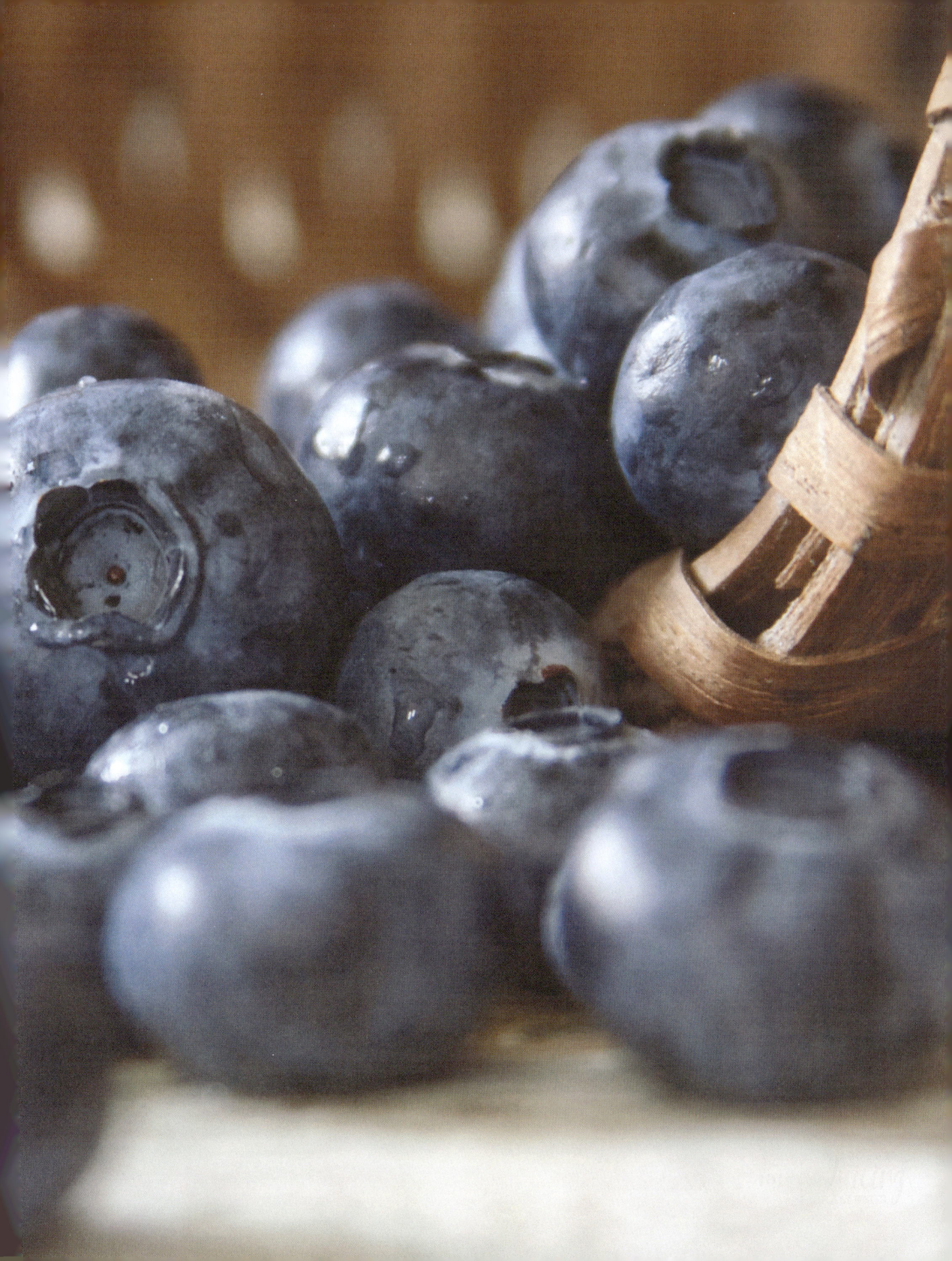

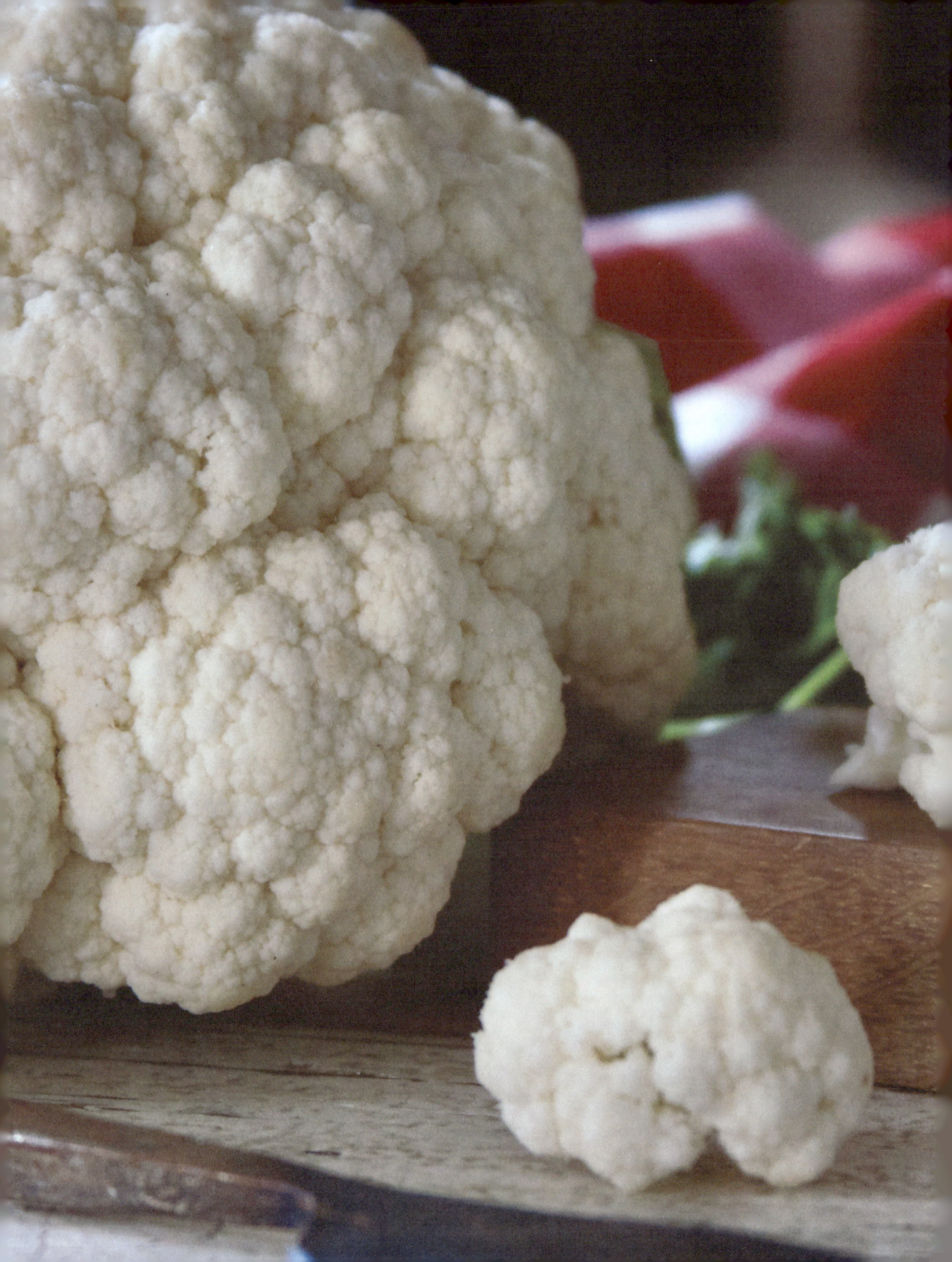

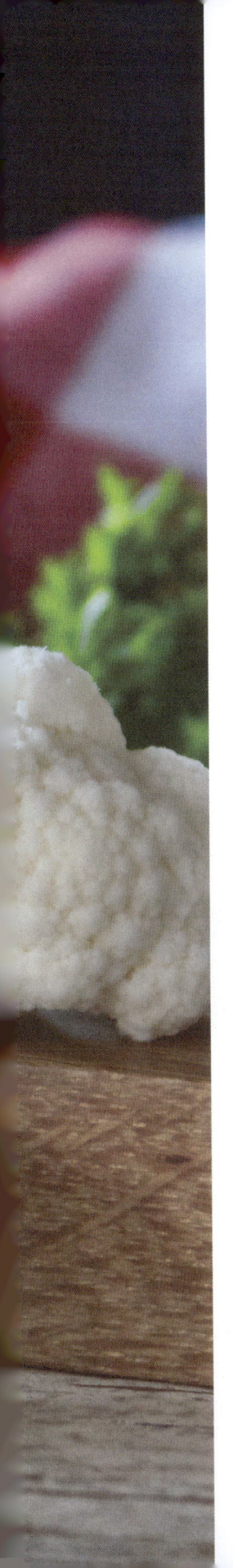

## O

**Onion** — Garlic, leeks, shallot
**Orange** — Grapefruit, clementine, tangerine, kiwi, mango, papaya
**Oregano** — Sage

## P

**Parsley** — Cilantro, kale, arugula
**Parsnip** — Turnip, parsley root, carrot
**Peaches** — Nectarines, plums, apple, pear
**Pear** — Apple, peach, plum
**Pineapple** — Orange grapefruit, mango
**Pomegranate** — Pineapple, strawberries
**Pumpkin** — Sweet potato, butternut squash, acorn squash

## Q

**Quinoa** — Brown rice, cooked barley, cooked couscous, garbanzo beans (chickpeas)

## R

**Radish** — Red cabbage, tomato
**Raisins** — Dried cranberries, figs
**Red/purple cabbage** — Green cabbage, radish, cauliflower, broccoli
**Romaine** — Spinach, bib lettuce, radicchio, endive, Boston lettuce, green or red leaf lettuce
**Rosemary** — Thyme, marjoram, caraway seed, dried rosemary, savory

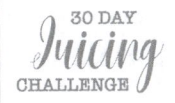

## S

**Shallot** — Garlic, onion

**Spinach** — Kale, chard, romaine lettuce, collard greens

**Strawberries** — Raspberries, blackberries, cherries

**Summer squash** — Zucchini, cucumber, celery

**Swiss chard** — Kale, spinach, romaine, mustard/collard/beet/turnip greens, green cabbage, arugula, watercress

## T

**Tangerine** — Orange, grapefruit

**Thyme** — Rosemary

**Tomato** — Radish, red pepper, watermelon

**Turmeric root** — Powdered turmeric, saffron, curry powder, ginger

## W

**Watermelon** — Red grapefruit, cantaloupe, honeydew, tomato, radish

**White wine vinegar** — Red wine vinegar, raw apple cider vinegar or lemon

## Z

**Zucchini** — Celery, cucumber, summer squash

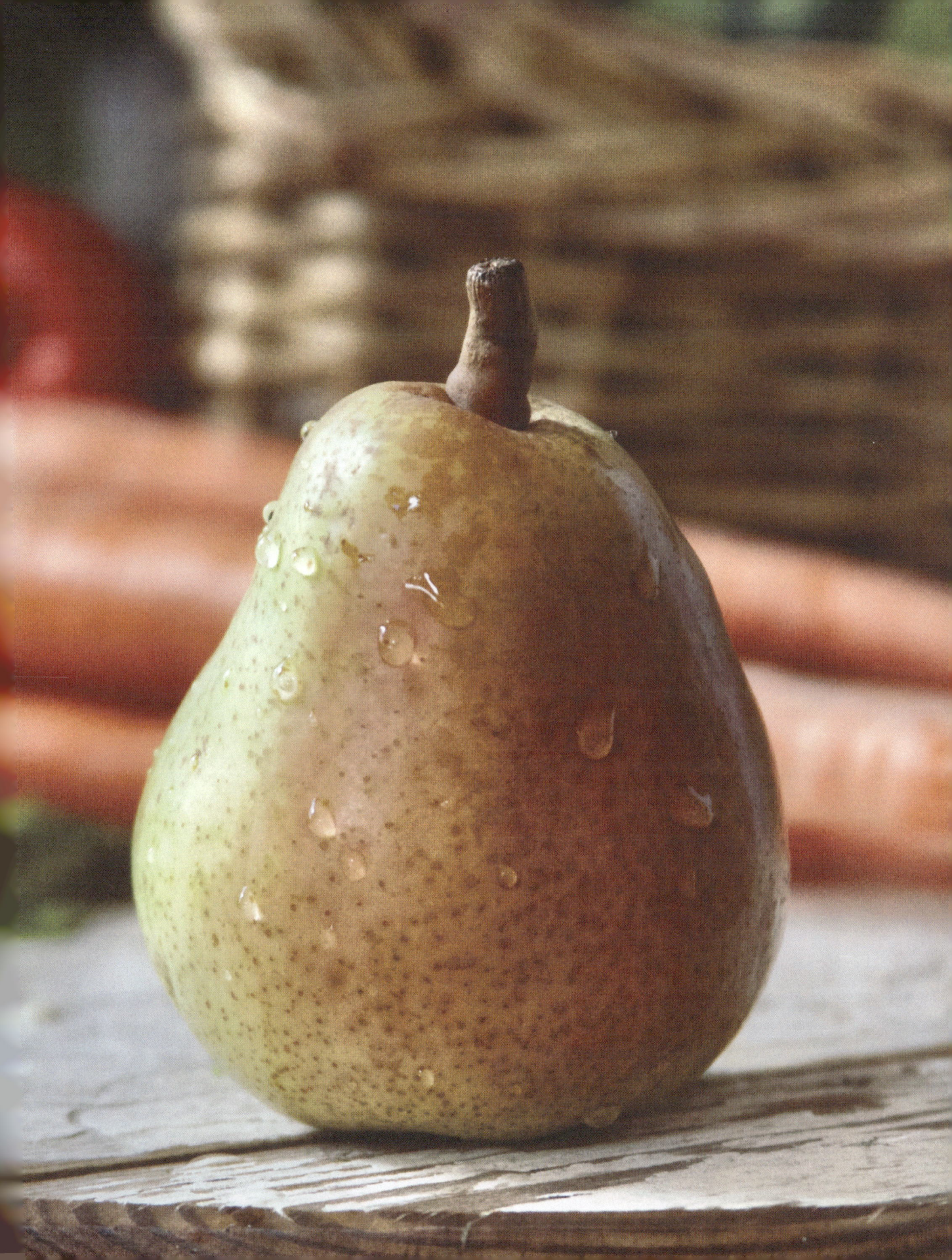

# RESOURCES

2013 Oct;22(10):1295-303. doi: 10.1517/13543784.2013.825249. Epub 2013 Aug 1.Curcumin: a novel therapeutic for burn pain and wound healing.

American Heart Association's diet and lifestyle recommendations. (2017, March 27)

British Journal of Nutrition, Volume 111, Issue 1. 14 January 2014 , pp. 1-11.

Cardiology. 1987;74 Suppl 1:12-9.Mechanism of vasodilation by nitrates: role of cyclic GMP.

Cheppudira B1, Fowler M, McGhee L, Greer A, Mares A, Petz L, Devore D, Loyd DR, Clifford JL.

Cholesterol-lowering effects of dietary fiber: a meta-analysis. Am J Clin Nutr. 1999 Jan;69(1):30-42.

Curr Top Med Chem. 2011;11(14):1752-66.Dietary antioxidants: immunity and host defense. Puertollano MA1, Puertollano E, de Cienfuegos GÁ, de Pablo MA.

Br J Nutr. 2012 Dec 14;108(11):2066-74. doi: 10.1017/S0007114512000190. Epub 2012 Mar 14.Blood pressure-lowering effects of beetroot juice and novel beetroot-enriched bread products in normotensive male subjects.

Foods That Heal: A Guide to Understanding and Using the Healing Powers of Natural Foods, Dr. Bernard Jensen.

Glycemic index and glycemic load for 100+ foods. (Aug 27, 2015.) Retrieved from: https://www.health.harvard.edu/diseases-and-conditions/glycemic-index-and-glycemic-load-for-100-foods.

Gollwitzer, P. M. (1993). Goal achievement: The role of intentions. In W. Stroebe & M. Hewstone (Eds.), European review of social psychology (Vol. 4, pp. 141-185). Chichester, UK: Wiley.

Halliwell B, Gutteridge JMC. Free radicals in biology and medicine. 4th. Oxford, UK: Clarendon Press; 2007.

Heinerman's New Encyclopedia of Fruits & Vegetables (Revised & Expanded) Heinerman, John. 1995.

Hobbs DA1, Kaffa N, George TW, Methven L, Lovegrove JA.

Ir J Med Sci. 2017 Nov;186(4):895-902. doi: 10.1007/s11845-016-1551-2. Epub 2017 Jan 3.Nitrate-rich beetroot juice selectively lowers ambulatory pressures and LDL cholesterol in uncontrolled but not controlled hypertension: a pilot study.

Kameya H, Watanabe J, Takano-Ishikawa Y, et al. Comparison of scavenging capacities of vegetables by ORAC and EPR. Food Chemistry, Volume 145, 15 February 2014, pages 866-873.

Kerley CP1,2,3, Dolan E4, Cormican L5.

Kidney health: Citric acid and kidney stones. (n.d.) uwhealth.org/healthfacts/nutrition/353.html

Kim SY, Yoon S, Kwon SM, et al. Kale Juice Improves Coronary Artery Disease Risk Factors in Hypercholesterolemic Men. Biomedical and Environmental Sciences, Volume 21, Issue 2, February 2008, pages 91-97.

Konsue N, Ioannides C. Modulation of carcinogen-metabolising cytochromes P450 in human liver by the chemopreventive phytochemical phenethyl isothiocyanate, a constituent of cruciferous vegetables. Toxicology. 2010 Feb 9;268(3):184-90. 2010.

Kukovetz WR, Holzmann S, Romanin C.

Li Y, Schellhorn HE. New developments and novel therapeutic perspectives for vitamin C. Critical Review. J. Nutr. 2007.

Life Sciences, Volume 116, Issue 1, 22 October 2014, Pages 1-7, Curcumin as a wound healing agent.

Pham-Huy NLA, He H, Pham-Huy C. Green tea and health. An overview. J. Food Agric. Environ. (JFAE) 2008.

Phytother Res. 2014 Jan;28(1):55-61. doi: 10.1002/ptr.4951. Epub 2013 Mar 1.Evaluation of the effect of beetroot juice on DMBA-induced damage in liver and mammary gland of female Sprague-Dawley rats.

Planta Med. 1998 May;64(4):353-6.Influence of piperine on the pharmacokinetics of curcumin in animals and human volunteers. Shoba G1, Joy D, Joseph T, Majeed M, Rajendran R, Srinivas PS.

Szaefer H1, Krajka-Kuźniak V, Ignatowicz E, Adamska T, Baer-Dubowska W.

The 150 Healthiest Foods on Earth: The Surprising, Unbiased Truth About What You Should Eat and Why, Bowden, Jonny. 2007.

University of Maryland Medical Center. Omega-3 fatty acids. Overview. 2007.

Valko M, Izakovic M, Mazur M, Rhodes CJ, et al. Role of oxygen radicals in DNA damage and cancer incidence. Mol. Cell Biochem. 2004.

Vegetables, Herbs and Fruit: An Illustrated Encyclopedia. Matthew Biggs, Jekka McVicar,Bob Flowerdew, 2013.

Willcox JK, Ash SL, Catignani GL. Antioxidants and prevention of chronic disease. Review. Crit. Rev. Food. Sci. Nutr. 2004.

Zaini, R., Clench, M. R., & Le Maitre, C. L. (2011, November). Bioactive chemicals from carrot (Daucus carota) juice extracts for the treatment of leukemia. Journal of Medicinal Food, 14(11), 1303-12.

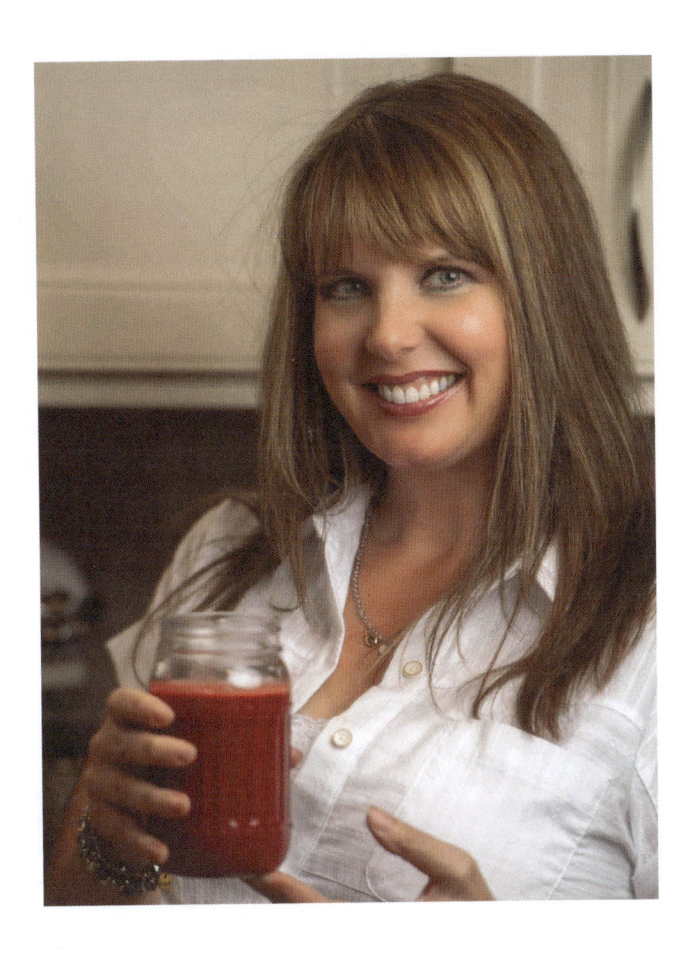

# About the Author

Tracee Sloan is known and loved all over the world for helping people reach for better health using the power of plants. Years of studying and experimenting with flavor combinations have resulted in her creating a variety of juice recipes that replenish vitamins and minerals while tasting delicious.

Nearly 20 years ago, Tracee's own health took a dramatic turn for the worse. With help from friends and family, she was able to heal herself with juicing, herbs and healthy food. Juicing became a way of life, and she began to inspire others to achieve their own long term health goals.

People from all over the globe have reached out to Tracee, sharing their stories of how juicing has helped them lose weight and take their lives back. Her message is simple: One positive change can lead to another, and another -- until soon your days are filled with healthy habits that are as natural as breathing.

First we make our habits,
*then our habits make us.*

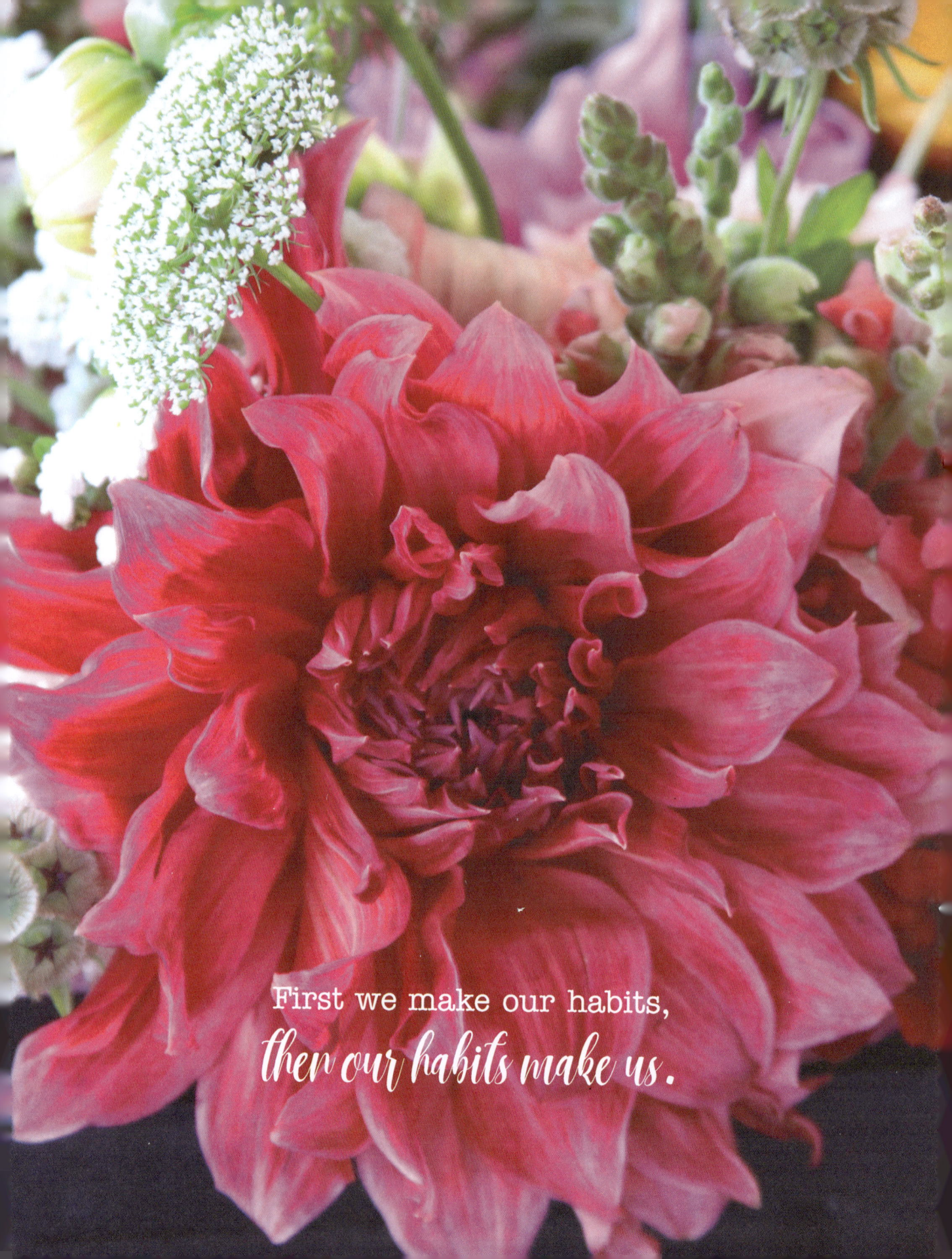

Printed in Great Britain
by Amazon